Ricardo Petroni

Role of Hypertonic Saline Solution in Lung Remodeling in Sepsis

Ricardo Petroni

Role of Hypertonic Saline Solution in Lung Remodeling in Sepsis

Could this be a potential therapy for septic patients?

ScienciaScripts

Imprint

Cover image: www.ingimage.com

This book is a translation from the original published under ISBN 978-3-330-76886-4.

Publisher:
Sciencia Scripts
is a trademark of
Dodo Books Indian Ocean Ltd. and OmniScriptum S.R.L publishing group

120 High Road, East Finchley, London, N2 9ED, United Kingdom
Str. Armeneasca 28/1, office 1, Chisinau MD-2012, Republic of Moldova, Europe
Managing Directors: Ieva Konstantinova, Victoria Ursu
info@omniscriptum.com

Printed at: see last page
ISBN: 978-620-8-60073-0

SUMMARY

DEDICATION

To my parents for all their support, teachings and understanding, without which this thesis would not have been possible.

THANKS

To Professor Francisco Garcia Soriano for his guidance, support, trust, dedication and friendship, which were essential to the completion of this thesis.

To my parents and my brothers Rosana, Reinaldo, Renan and Rodrigo for all their support and understanding.

To my grandparents, uncles and cousins who are always present in my life.

To Denise, Hermes and Suely, who took me in when I was still an undergraduate and were my great teachers, playing a fundamental role in the completion of this thesis.

To Thais, who, in addition to her friendship and teaching, made this thesis much more enjoyable.

To Ester and Vivian for always being willing to help, for their companionship and friendship.

To Professors Dr. Heraldo Possolo de Souza and Dr. Irineu Tadeu Velasco, for their suggestions that contributed to this thesis.

To Dr. Paolo Biselli for his immense contribution in carrying out the experiments and for discussing the results obtained.

To the friends and staff of LIM-51: Geraldo, Kelli and Fàtima, who helped directly with this thesis.

To the friends and students of LIM-51: Rosangela, Clara, Joleen, Isabela, Anne, Vanessa, Mariana Macedo, Mariana Maldonado, Mariana Theobaldo, Darkiane, Graça, Luis and all the others who have passed through the lab, for all their help.

To FAPESP for financial support

"Something is only impossible until someone doubts it and proves otherwise"

Albert Einstein

SUMMARY

Summary

Petroni, RC. Role of hypertonic saline solution (NaCl 7.5%) in pulmonary remodeling of endotoxemia induced by lipopolysaccharides. [thesis] São Paulo: School of Medicine, University of São Paulo; 2013.

Sepsis is an inappropriate inflammatory response triggered by the presence of bacteria and/or bacterial products such as Hpopolysaccharides (LPS). Severe sepsis and septic shock are associated with mortality rates of 40 to 60%. Respiratory failure is among the most frequent complications of severe sepsis, occurring in almost 80% of cases. Around 40% of patients with sepsis develop acute respiratory distress syndrome (ARDS), characterized mainly by altered respiratory function, the appearance of interstitial pulmonary edema and the deposition of collagen in the lungs. Although volume replacement is normally used in septic patients, there is no consensus on the volume to be administered, and the use of small volumes is currently recommended. In this context, hypertonic saline (7.5% NaCl, HS) has been presented as a potential therapeutic agent. In order to contribute to the knowledge of the benefits of hypertonic saline (HS) in sepsis, this study aimed to evaluate the action of early and late treatment with hypertonic saline on the lungs of endotoxemic rats. Wistar rats were separated into 4 groups (n=10): CTL (without any insult or treatment); LPS (injected with LPS 10mg/Kg i.p); HIPER (animals that received treatment with hypertonic solution 7.5% NaCl i.p at a dose of 4ml/Kg 15 min. or 1.5 hours after LPS injection) and SALINE (animals treated with saline 0.9% NaCl i.p. at a dose of 34ml/Kg 15 min. or 1.5 hours after LPS injection). Mortality was assessed, and after 24 hours pulmonary edema and mechanics, type I and type III collagens, MMP-9 expression and activity, FAK expression and nitric oxide (NO) synthesis. Our results showed that early treatment with hypertonic saline prevented the death of endotoxemic animals. None of the treatments modulated the inflammatory mediators. Early treatment with hypertonic saline decreased the synthesis of iNOS and nitrite, the expression and activity of MMP-9 and FAK, along with the deposition of type I collagen, preventing the replacement of collagen III. We observed an improvement in respiratory mechanics parameters. The late treatment with hypertonic solution did not show the same promising results as the early treatment, suggesting that the time of administration of hypertonic solution is of great importance for obtaining its therapeutic effects.

Keywords: Sepsis; Acute lung injury; Inflammation; Hypertonic saline solution; Pulmonary fibrosis; Adult respiratory distress syndrome; Collagen; Endotoxemia; Lipopolysaccharides; Rats.

INTRODUCTION

1. Introduction

1.1 - Sepsis: Clinic and Epidemiology

Sepsis is a clinical syndrome resulting from complications of serious infections and is characterized by a systemic inflammatory response and diffuse tissue damage. It is associated with a disruption of the normal inflammatory response, with massive and uncontrolled release of inflammatory mediators, creating a chain of events that lead to tissue damage (1-3).

Sepsis is a subgroup of the systemic inflammatory response syndrome (SIRS). It is defined as a systemic response to infection. It is manifested by the presence of two or more symptoms: a) a change in temperature, above 38° C or below 36° C; b) an increase in heart rate above 90 beats per minute; c) an increase in respiratory rate above 20 breaths per minute or pCO_2 below 32 mmHg and d) a blood leukocyte count above 12000/mm^3 or below 4000/mm^3 (4-6).

Approximately 70% of patients admitted to intensive care units (ICUs) develop systemic inflammatory response syndrome (SIRS), which can also occur in association with non-infectious events, such as polytrauma, surgery, pancreatitis and burns (7-9). When septic shock sets in, with systemic arterial hypotension that is difficult to control, this state can progress to multiple organ and system failure (7, 9-11). Gram-positive and Gram-negative bacteria are responsible for the majority of sepsis cases (36% and 35%, respectively). Severe sepsis and septic shock are associated with mortality rates of 40 to 60% (12). Data from the United States indicates that there are approximately 751,000 cases of sepsis per year (9, 13). Sepsis, SIRS and septic shock together represent the most important cause of death in adult ICUs, surpassing cardiovascular diseases (14).

In Brazil, data from the BASES study showed that sepsis is the main cost generator in the public and private sectors (15). Spending on ICU patients in 2003 amounted to R$17.34 billion, which represents approximately 30 to 35% of total healthcare spending. A study published in 2006 in Brazilian intensive care units showed that 16.7% of ICU patients developed sepsis, severe sepsis or septic shock, with a mortality rate of 16.7% for patients with sepsis, 34.4% for patients with severe sepsis and 65.3% for patients with septic shock (15-17).

Mortality has not changed in the last two decades despite the development of new antibiotics and the improvement of intensive treatment measures (7, 9, 10, 18). New strategies for treating sepsis have focused on endotoxin inhibitors (anti-endotoxin antibody), cytokine inhibitors (TNF) and blockers of vasoactive substance production (nitric oxide) (19). Despite considerable investment in new drugs, most of them have not shown any benefit in reducing mortality in clinical trials. Studies of early hemodynamic intervention directed by venous oxygen saturation have been shown to be possible therapies for reducing mortality in this pathology (20-22).

1.2 - Pathophysiology of Sepsis and Systemic Inflammatory Response Syndrome (SIRS)

Sepsis, the systemic response to infection, is mediated by cytokines produced by inflammatory cells, which stimulate specific receptors on immune system cells and target organs. The cytokines: interleukin 1 beta (IL-1β), interleukin 6 (IL-6), interleukin 8 (IL-8) and tumor necrosis factor-α (TNF-α) are early triggers in this process (2326). These cytokines stimulate the release of other inflammatory response mediators such as arachidonic acid-derived products (PGE2, TXA2), platelet-activating factor (PAF); vasoactive peptides such as bradykinin, angiotensin, vasoactive intestinal peptide; a variety of complement-derived products, as well as other cytokines (12).

1.3 - Molecular Mechanisms of LPS Action

The Hpopolysaccharide (LPS) present in the wall of Gram-negative bacteria is an important tool in the study of sepsis and is normally used as a study model for lung diseases resulting from sepsis (27-30).

The LPS of several gram-negative microbial families is made up of a polysaccharide portion covalently linked to lipid A (LA). The outer membrane of the bacteria has the O chain which is characteristic and unique to each bacterial serotype and the LA which represents the endotoxic principle of the LPS (31). After LPS enters the bloodstream, at least two proteins, LBP and CD14, compete to bind to this toxic macromolecule. The binding of LPS to serum LBP facilitates the transfer of LPS to CD14. After association with serum factors, LPS interacts with receptors expressed by the endotoxin's target cells, such as granulocytes, lymphocytes, endothelial cells and, in particular, monocytes/macrophages (23-26).

CD14 is a protein on the outer surface of the monocyte cell membrane that facilitates LPS-induced cell activation. CD14 together with the MD2 protein participate in the presentation of LPS to the Toll-like receptor type 4 (TLR4), subsequently activating leukocytes to secrete cytokines and initiating an acute inflammatory response (Figure 1) (32).

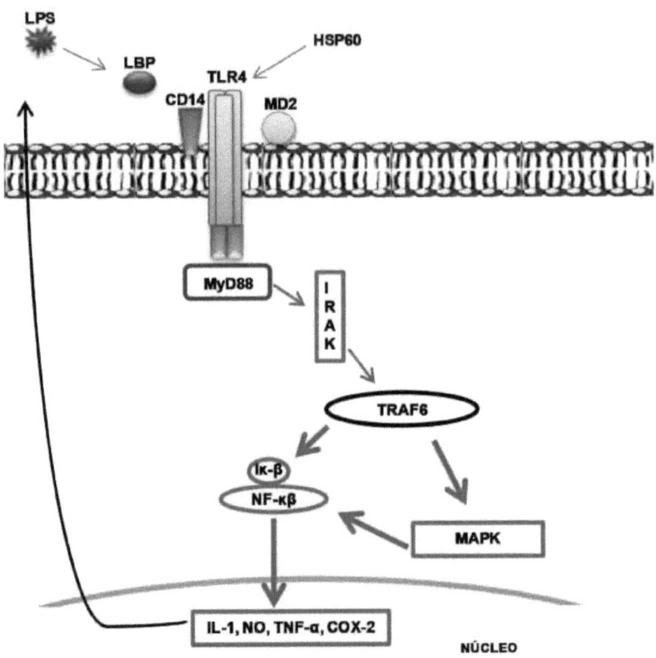

Figure 1. Cell signaling pathways triggered by LPS.

1.4 - Inflammatory Mediators

The central event in the pathophysiological cascade of sepsis is an excessive systemic release of pro-inflammatory cytokines such as TNF-α, interleukin (IL)-1, IL-6, IL-12, IL-18 and interferon-γ in response to LPS (33).

These cytokines activate cellular systems (phagocytes and endothelium) and humoral systems (coagulation pathways and complement activation, low molecular weight mediators) which are primarily geared towards eliminating invading bacteria and can cause generalized self-destructive inflammation and lead to multiple organ failure (34).

Cytokines promote the recruitment of leukocytes to the inflammatory site, as well as their activation with a consequent increase in microbicidal activity, the local response being fundamental for controlling the infection. The progression from a localized infection to a systemic condition is characterized by the presence of pro-inflammatory cytokines in the circulation and the activation of circulating cells, as well as the presence of bacteria, endotoxins or exotoxins. These cytokines play an important role in the development of sepsis, interfering in the prognosis, evolution and intensity of tissue damage (35).

The immune system has a wide range of cells and substances at its disposal to protect against infectious agents. Various cell types such as monocytes, macrophages, lymphocytes, neutrophils and endothelial cells participate in the exacerbated inflammatory response in sepsis by releasing a wide variety of mediators (36). Monocytes and macrophages release pro-inflammatory cytokines such as TNF-α and IL-1β. T lymphocytes can have two polarizations: T helper 1 (Th1) and T helper 2 (Th2). The Th1 pattern is characterized by the secretion of IFN-γ, TNF-α, IL-12 and in the Th2 pattern there is the release of IL-4 and IL-10.

TNF-α is the first cytokine released by monocytes and macrophages in response to endotoxin. It is responsible for increasing the procoagulant activity of vascular epithelial cells, neutrophil activation, as well as increasing the activation of adhesion molecules, leading to tissue damage (37). The cytokine IL-10 has anti-inflammatory activity. It is synthesized by Th2 cells such as monocytes and B lymphocytes. Its function is to inhibit the secretion of pro-inflammatory cytokines by macrophages, protecting the host from the systemic inflammatory response induced by endotoxins (37).

In addition to these mediators, acute phase proteins, activation of the coagulation system, the complement system and increased nitric oxide production are related to the deleterious effects of sepsis in both patients and experimental models (38).

1.5 - Lung and Sepsis

The first organ affected in intra-abdominal sepsis is the lung (5). Respiratory failure is among the most frequent complications of severe sepsis, occurring in almost 80% of cases, but the mechanisms of acute pulmonary failure in sepsis are still not fully understood (32, 39-41).

Studies analyzing organ dysfunction and death in patients with sepsis of abdominal origin found that 28% of patients had respiratory failure, and 63% of them died (39).

Acute lung injury in septic patients is characterized by neutrophilic infiltration and increased alveolar capillary permeability caused by neutrophil adhesion to the pulmonary capillaries (1).

Sepsis causes damage to the pulmonary vascular endothelium secondary to inflammation which produces progressive interstitial edema, leading to an imbalance between ventilation and pulmonary perfusion, with refractory hypoxemia, decreased lung compliance, deposition of fibronectin and collagen causing the need for mechanical ventilation for adequate tissue oxygenation. As the septic condition progresses, mixed venous oxygen saturation increases and the arteriovenous difference decreases (27). The alveolar-arterial gradient widens and there is a decrease in the partial pressure of oxygen in arterial blood (pO_2) (39-42).

Neutrophil activation and excessive release of cytotoxic mediators in sepsis can cause intense damage to lung tissue, contributing to post-traumatic complications such as acute respiratory distress syndrome (ARDS) and multiple organ failure (43).

1.6 - Pulmonary Fibrosis

Patients with sepsis-induced ARDS have decreased lung compliance, thus increasing respiratory work and requiring assisted ventilation. This may be due to the development of pulmonary fibrosis, thus altering lung compliance and consequently lung functions (44, 45). During ARDS, fibroblasts proliferate in the lung interstitium and new collagen is deposited there (46).

Pulmonary fibrosis in this disease is often defined as interstitial, as the structures between the air spaces appear enlarged by fibrotic material. Fibrosis usually results from adverse collapses of intra-alveolar fibrosis in which edema and cellular debris from the oxidative stage of the disease are incorporated into the alveolar wall (47).

Fibrotic lung diseases are characterized by the expansion of the mesenchymal cell population and the deposition of collagen in late periods. However, recently several studies have shown that, contrary to what was thought, collagen deposition in lung tissue occurs early (40, 48, 49). Marshall et al. showed in their study that fibroproliferation occurred in the early stages of ARDS, suggesting that the mechanisms that trigger collagen deposition (fibroblast proliferation and pro-collagen synthesis) are rapidly triggered in this disease (27). Studies have shown that patients with ARDS resulting from sepsis who survived more than two weeks had twice as much collagen in their lungs. This may have contributed to the progressive loss of respiratory function shown by these patients (50, 51). These changes have recently been shown to be a consequence of the activation of focal adhesion *kinase* (FAK) (52). FAK is a protein in the cytoskeleton and/or cell membrane, which transduces signals resulting from inflammation or tension in lung tissue. FAK activation leads to cell activation and consequently collagen production, which will result in damage to the lung architecture, altering its compliance and gas exchange (53, 54). Studies have shown that the activation of FAK in lung tissue is responsible for the excessive deposition of collagen in the tissue, leading to a decrease in respiratory function (55, 56).

The synthesis of collagen in the lung is a dynamic process, necessary to maintain the architecture of the tissue. Collagen fibers are the main components of the extracellular matrix (ECM). Despite the abundant presence of various types of collagen in connective tissues, type I, II, III (fibrillar) and IV, V and VI (non-fibrillar) collagens represent the main collagen fibers. The lung is characterized by the presence mainly of type I collagen (most abundant in lung tissue), type III collagen and type V collagen (57).

. Deaths caused by ARDS occur when fibrosis plays a predominant role in healing, resulting in a worsening of lung compliance and tissue oxygenation. Excessive collagen synthesis in the lung and its accumulation in the advanced stages of the disease can contribute to the high death rates of patients and promote progressive and intense respiratory dysfunction (27).

1.7 - Metalloproteinases (MMPs)

Pulmonary fibrosis is characterized by the accumulation of extracellular matrix proteins, including collagen. The imbalance between the synthesis and degradation of extracellular matrix proteins leads to the accumulation of collagen in the tissue. Activated neutrophils present during ARDS release enzymes such as metalloproteinases responsible for tissue invasion and for controlling the deposition of extracellular matrix proteins.

+ Metalloproteinases (MMPs) are $Ca^{(2+)}$and Zn^{2}-dependent endopeptidases responsible for digesting various structural components of the extracellular matrix (ECM), such as collagen, elastin, fibronectin and laminin. MMPs can also digest other extracellular proteins. Their targets include a large number of cell surface receptors, growth factors, cytokines and chemokines (58). Proteolysis triggered by the action of MMPs plays an important role in various biological processes such as embryonic development, morphogenesis, bone remodeling, homeostasis, healing, etc. The expression and activity of MMPs are strictly regulated and controlled by the action of endogenous mechanisms such as tissue inhibitors of MMPs (TIMPs) (59). Studies have shown that alterations in the balance during this regulation result in a wide variety of diseases such as tumors and multiple sclerosis (60, 61).

More than 27 MMPs have been identified in humans, which are grouped into collagenases, gelatinases, stromelysins, matrilysins and membrane MMPs (60). MMPs are secreted by various cells (fibroblasts, epithelial cells, macrophages) as latent proenzymes (zymogen), which need to be activated in the extracellular environment by breaking the zinc bond in their active center, through physical, chemical or proteolytic processes. This cleavage of the secreted enzyme's prepeptide can be activated by the action of proteolytic enzymes from other families as well as by the MMPs themselves (62). MMP-9 is particularly important in tissue infiltration by polymorphonuclear cells during inflammation, since they can degrade components of the vascular basement membrane, such as types I, II, IV and V collagens, as well as fibronectin and gelatin(63). The potential destructive activity of metalloproteinases is limited by IL-10, which not only inhibits the production of MMP-9, but also induces the production of TIMPs. Various cytokines such as IFN-γ, IL-4 and TGF-β decrease the production of MMPs. However, IL-1 β and TNF- α increase the timing and secretion of these enzymes (64).

1.8 - Nitric Oxide

Nitric oxide (NO) is a free radical synthesized from L-arginine. The enzymes that catalyze this reaction are called NO synthase (NOS). There are three different isoforms of NOS in mammalian cells: endothelial NOS (eNOS or NOS3) found in endothelial cells, epithelial cells and cardiac myocytes; neuronal NOS (nNOS or NOS1) found in neuronal cells and skeletal muscle; inducible NOS (iNOS or NOS2) found in macrophages, hepatocytes and lung epithelial cells (65-68).

eNOS and nNOS are constitutively expressed enzymes and their activation is dependent on an increase in intracellular Ca^{2+}. eNOS is involved in regulating vascular tone while nNOS plays an important role in neurotransmission. iNOS is functionally independent of Ca^{2+} and is not normally expressed constitutively, but its expression is induced in certain pathophysiological events and in the immune response (67, 68). iNOS is expressed by pro-inflammatory stimuli such as endotoxin (LPS) and gamma interferon (IFN-γ). The NO produced by iNOS plays an important role in the protective effect exerted by macrophages against bacteria (65).

Under physiological conditions, NO plays a cytoprotective role by eliminating free radicals such as superoxide, limiting their cytotoxic effect on lung tissue (69). In sepsis, NO has a toxic product profile, promoting an intense immunoregulatory process through the activation of neutrophils, macrophages, monocytes and endothelial cells (67). In experimental models of endotoxemia, the lungs express extremely high levels of iNOS in alveolar macrophages, epithelial cells, endothelial cells and pulmonary interstitial cells for prolonged periods. These high levels of iNOS are among the main causes of lung damage resulting from endotoxemia (65, 69).

1.9 - Volume resuscitation

The inflammatory response resulting from sepsis leads to an increase in water loss and worsening of microvascular permeability, resulting in a decrease in intravascular volume and the need for volume replacement in order to achieve and maintain adequate tissue perfusion pressure (70, 71).

Volume replacement is an important treatment for endotoxemic shock. Studies have shown that volume replacement improves hemodynamic parameters, restores intravascular volume, improves perfusion and reduces tissue damage resulting from sepsis (72, 73). Although volume replacement is normally used in septic patients, there is no consensus on the volume to be administered. Studies show that patients treated with a positive fluid balance have worse clinical results, such as reduced lung function, increased intra-abdominal pressure and an increased risk of mortality (74, 75).

The administration of smaller volumes of fluids to patients with ARDS is responsible for the patient's improvement, reducing the time spent on mechanical ventilation without any associated morbidity (74).

1.10 - Hypertonic Solution - NaCl 7.5% (HS)

Hypertonic saline (7.5% saline, HS) has been shown to be a potential therapeutic agent in various injury models (76). The use of HS has shown inhibition of acute lung injury (ALI) caused by ischemia- reperfusion, hemorrhagic shock and acute pancreatitis in experimental models (43, 76).

Velasco et al. (77) observed in 1980 that resuscitation with hypertonic saline in dogs induced by hemorrhagic shock was very effective in restoring the hemodynamic parameters of these animals. Recently, other authors have shown that HS is an alternative form of resuscitation, with great immunomodulatory potential in trauma victims and patients with sepsis (39, 78-80). Hypertonic saline (HS) has been shown to have beneficial effects as a volume-restoring fluid in the clinical scenario (8185). The use of HS has been linked to significant changes in innate immunity, altering neutrophil activation, inhibiting the oxidative *burst*, attenuating the cytotoxic response in neutrophils and inhibiting monocyte/macrophage activation *in vitro* (86, 87).

In addition to increasing plasma volume, HS has significant anti-inflammatory effects (88). Hypertonic saline favorably modulates cellular events in patients with SIRS (89), inhibiting the expression of TNF-α and increasing the production of IL-10 by alveolar macrophages, playing a protective role in relation to the systemic inflammatory response (90). Another important role of HS is related to the reduction of inflammatory infiltrate, reduction of pulmonary inflammation and reduction of interleukin 6 (IL-6) levels in lung tissue of animals that received volume replacement (91, 92). The presence of neutrophils in lung tissue, which plays an important role in the mechanism of tissue damage, is also attenuated by the use of

HS in various models of acute lung injury (43, 93, 94).

The accumulation of neutrophils in the lung is a necessary prerequisite for the development of lung damage (91). Hypertonic saline reduces, but does not abolish, the pro-inflammatory pathways, allowing an adequate balance between pro- and anti-inflammatory cytokines, thus maintaining the ability to eliminate bacteria efficiently and reducing disseminated inflammation (80). Data on the immunoregulatory potential of hypertonic saline to reduce the inflammatory response, in addition to the classic hemodynamic effects, point to the possibility of an appropriate therapeutic action in patients with sepsis. The search for therapies that interfere with the inflammatory and immunological response in inflammatory processes with a high mortality rate, such as ARDS resulting from sepsis, could mean important advances in the treatment of patients with these pathologies.

OBJECTIVES

2. Objectives

2.1 - General Objective:

The aim of this study was to demonstrate the therapeutic action of treatment with hypertonic saline solution early and late on the pathophysiological mechanisms that produce pulmonary alterations in endotoxemia induced by lipopolysaccharide.

2.2 - Specific Objectives:

To study the effects of early and late treatment with hypertonic solution and saline solution on:

- Pulmonary edema in endotoxemic rats.
- The inflammatory process in the lung tissue of endotoxemic rats.
- The remodeling of lung tissue through the analysis of collagen deposition and the expression and activity of MMP-9.
- Functional lung mechanics.
- The focal adhesion protein kinase (FAK) signaling pathway and its possible relationship with nitric oxide synthase in endotoxemic rat lungs.

METHODS

3. Methods

3.1 - Biological Model

Male Wistar rats weighing between 200-250 grams were selected from the Central Bioterium of the Medical School of the University of São Paulo. The rats were kept in cages for seven days, in a room with a controlled temperature and light cycle, receiving water and food *ad libitum*. During the experiment, the animals remained in the Maintenance Bioterium of LIM 17 - Rheumatology Discipline, under the responsibility of biologist Antônio dos Santos Filho.

All procedures were carried out in accordance with the standards established by the Brazilian College of Animal Experimentation (COBEA) and *The Universities Federation for Animals Welfare* (UFAW). Our project was approved by the Research Ethics Committee of the Hospital das Clinicas of the Medical School of the University of São Paulo (CAPPesq). Research protocol no·0428/09.

3.2 - Anesthesia

To treat the animals with injections of hypertonic saline or saline and for the thoracotomy and lung removal process, the animals were anaesthetized with 3% halothane in a gas mixture of 30% oxygen and 70% nitrous oxide.

3.3 - Study time

The tests were carried out 24 hours after the intraperitoneal injection of LPS and in the case of the treated animals there were groups that received hypertonic saline or saline 15 minutes (early) and groups that received hypertonic saline or saline 1.5 hours (late) after the injection of LPS.

3.4 - Group constitution and experimental protocol

Each group consists of 10 animals.

- **Control Group (CTL) 24 hours:**

The rats received no insult or treatment.

- **Endotoxemic Group (LPS) 24 hours:**

The rats were subjected to endotoxemia by intraperitoneal (i.p) injection at a dose of 10mg/Kg *of Lipopolysaccharide* (LPS) from *Escherichia coli* (serotype 026:B6/Sigma, MO, USA) (95). The animals were sacrificed 24 hours after treatment.

- **24-hour endotoxemic group treated with hypertonic solution (HIPER) 15 minutes or 1.5 hours after LPS injection:**

The animals submitted to endotoxemia by intraperitoneal (i.p.) injection at a dose of 10mg/Kg of LPS, received hypertonic saline (7.5% NaCl) at a dose of 4 ml/kg by injection into the penile vein 15 minutes (early) or 1.5 hours (late) after the LPS injection. The animals were sacrificed 24 hours after treatment.

- **24-hour endotoxemic group treated with saline solution (SALINA) 15 minutes or 1.5 hours after LPS injection:**

The animals submitted to endotoxemia by intraperitoneal (i.p.) injection at a dose of 10mg/Kg of LPS were given saline solution (0.9% NaCl) at a dose of 34 ml/kg by injection into the penile vein 15 minutes (early) or 1.5 hours (late) after the LPS injection. The animals were sacrificed 24 hours after treatment.

3.5 - Survival Curve

After injection of LPS and/or treatment with saline or hypertonic solution, the animals were observed and deaths were recorded every 12 hours for a total period of 72 hours.

3.6 - Determination of Pulmonary Edema

The lungs were removed from the animals, stored in 1.5 mL tubes and weighed immediately after removal. The lungs were stored in an oven for 48 hours and weighed again. The weight of the lung immediately after removal was divided by its dry weight (ratio), measured after 48 hours in the oven. The final result was corrected for the weight of each animal in order to minimize possible errors due to the variation in weight of these animals.

3.7 - Lung Function Analysis

The animals in each group were anesthetized with Sodium Pentobarbital (50 mg/kg, intraperitoneally), tracheostomized with a 20G intravascular catheter and connected to a small animal respirator (flexiVent, SCIREQ, Montreal, Canada). A schematic diagram of the mechanical respirator used is shown in Figure 2.

The animals were ventilated with a tidal volume of 8 mL/kg and a respiratory rate of 90 cycles/minute. We used a PEEP of 5 cmH_2O connected to the ventilator's expiratory valve.

Ptr (tracheal pressure), *v* (flow) and V (volume) were collected during a sinusoidal oscillation. The resistance (Rrs) and elastance (Ers) of the respiratory system were calculated automatically by a computer using the equation of motion:

Ptr(t)= Ers.V(t) + Rrs.*v*(t)

Where:

- Ptr (t) is the pressure at the air opening
- V(t) is the volume entering the lungs
- *v* (t) is the air flow
- (t) is the time

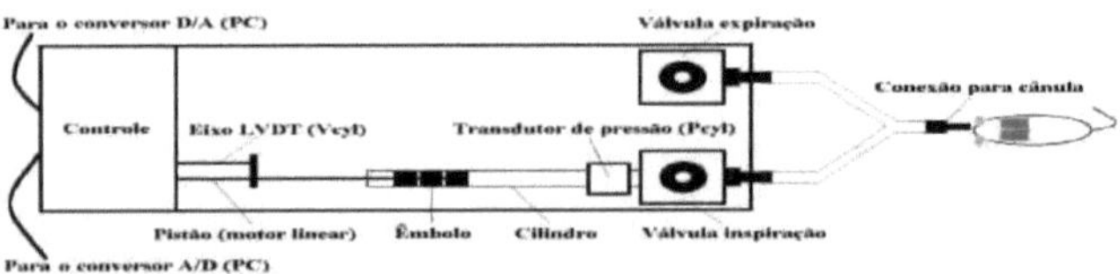

Figure 2 - Schematic of the small animal respirator (Flexivent-Scireq) used to collect respiratory mechanics data.

3.8 - Gene Expression Quantification

After thoracotomy and dissection, 100 mg of the right lung were removed, cleaned in 0.9% saline solution and stored in cryogenic tubes in a -80°C freezer. These tissues were homogenized using a stainless steel grater cooled with liquid nitrogen (Bel-Art Products, NJ, USA) and a ceramic pistil. The samples were stored in 1.5 mL tubes for RNA extraction.

3.8.1 - RNA extraction

Total RNA from the homogenates was extracted with 1 mL of Trizol (Invitrogen, CA, USA) in 1.5 mL tubes, followed by incubation for 5 minutes at room temperature. Then 200 µL of chloroform was added, the tubes were *vortexed* and incubated for 3 minutes at room temperature. After incubation, the samples were centrifuged (Eppendorf 5804R) at 4°C for 15 minutes at 12000g. The supernatant was transferred to another 1.5 mL tube, where 500 µL of ice-cold isopropanol was added. After incubating for 10 minutes, the sample was centrifuged again at 4°C for 10 minutes at 12000g. The supernatant was discarded and 1 mL of ice-cold 70% ethanol was added to the *pellet*, followed by centrifugation at 4°C for 5 minutes at 7500g. The supernatant was discarded and the *pellet* was reconstituted in 50 µL of water with 0.1% diethylpyrocarbonate (Sigma, MO, USA) and stored in a -80°C freezer.

3.8.2 - Real-time PCR reaction

Gene expression was assessed by real-time PCR using the StepOne Real-Time PCR System (Applied Biosystems, NY, USA) with the Platinum® SYBR® Green qPCR SuperMix

UDG kit (Invitrogen, CA, USA) which contains SYBR® Green I as a fluorophore. Quantification of gene expression was carried out by $2^{-\Delta\Delta C_T}$ (96, 97), using the β2M gene as an internal control. The sequences of the specific primers used, as well as the size of the fragments were:

β2M:sense CGTGATCTTTCTGGTGCTTGTC; antisense

TTCTGAATGGCAAGCACGAC, generating a product of 604 base pairs. The reaction consisted of 40 cycles and *an annealing* temperature 60°C.

iNOS: sense TGGAGCATCCCAAGTACGAGTG; antisense

GCCCATGTACCAACCATTGAAG, generating a product of 170 base pairs. The reaction consisted of 40 cycles and *an annealing* temperature 58°C.

MMP-9: sense CAAACCCTGCGTATTTCCAT; antisense

AGAGTACTGCTTGCCCAGGA, generating a 223 base pair product. The reaction consisted of 40 cycles and *an annealing* temperature 60°C.

3.9 - Analysis of Metalloproteinase-9 (MMP-9) Activity - Zymography

Samples of the collected tissues were homogenized in TX-100 lysis buffer (Triton X-100, 10% glycerol, 135mM NaCl, 20mM Tris pH8.0). The lysate samples were then centrifuged at 14000g for 10 minutes at 4°C. The supernatant was collected and the protein concentration quantified using the Bradford method. Samples of 5µg/ml of protein were added to sample buffer (2% SDS, 60mM Tris pH6.8, 30% glycerol and 0.01% bromophenol blue) and applied to a 10% polyacrylamide gel containing 0.2% gelatine. After electrophoresis, the gel was washed in 10mM Tris (pH 8.0) containing 2.5% Triton X-100 to remove the SDS and renature the proteins. The gel was then incubated for 15 minutes in developer buffer (50mM Tris pH8.8, 5mM $CaCl_2$, 0.02% NaN_3). The gel was then incubated for 72 hours at 37°C in developer solution only. The gel was stained with Coomassie Brilliant Blue R-250 (Amersham, NJ, USA) for 2 hours. It was then destained in a solution of 40% methanol and 10% glacial acetic acid in distilled water. MMPs are identified as clear lysis bands (88 kDa) on a blue background. Protein expression was analyzed by gel densitometry using the public domain program "*Image J*". The samples were normalized by the control (control = 1).

3.10 - Quantification of Cytokines - ELISA

The cytokines TNF-α and IL-10 were measured from lung tissue homogenate. Approximately 100mg of tissue was pulverized in liquid nitrogen. The material was homogenized in 1 ml of

TX- 100 lysis buffer (100mM Tris-HCL pH 7.5, 1% sodium deoxycholate, 1% Triton X- 100, 150mM NaCl, 0.1% SDS) plus protease inhibitors (1mg/ml pepstatin A, 100mM PMSF). The samples were then centrifuged at 14000g for 10 minutes at 4°C. The supernatant was collected and the protein concentration was quantified using the Bradford method (Bio-Rad, CA, USA). Measurements were made by ELISA, using a kit from R&D Systems (Minneapolis, MN, USA).

96-well plates were adsorbed with monoclonal anti-cytokine capture antibody of interest, diluted in PBS for 12 hours. The plates were then washed with a PBS solution containing 0.05% tween 20. The non-specific sites were blocked with PBS containing 1% BSA (bovine serum albumin - Sigma, MO, USA) for 1 hour. The plate was washed to remove the blocking solution. The samples and standards were then placed in the respective wells and incubated for 2 hours. At the end of the period, the plates were washed. The detection antibody, conjugated to peroxidase, was added and incubated for 2 hours. The plates were washed again. At the end of the washes, the peroxidase substrate, tetramethylbenzidine, was added and left to act for 15 to 20 minutes. The peroxidase-tetramethylbenzidine reaction generated a blue color. At the end of incubation, a stop solution (H2SO4 - 2N) was added, resulting in a yellow color. The optical density of each well was detected using a plate reader

SpectraMax™ Microplate Reader (Molecular devises, Minnesota, USA) at a wavelength of 450nm. Cytokine concentrations (pg/mL) were normalized by total protein concentrations.

3.11 - Protein Expression Analysis - Western Blot

Fragments of 100mg of tissue were pulverized in liquid nitrogen. The material was homogenized in TX-100 lysis buffer (100mM Tris-HCL pH 7.5, 1% sodium deoxycholate, 1% Triton X-100, 150mM NaCl, 0.1% SDS) plus protease inhibitors (1mg/ml pepstatin A, 100mM PMSF). The samples were then centrifuged at 14000g for 10 minutes at 4°C. The supernatant was collected and the protein concentration was quantified using the Bradford method (Bio-Rad, CA, USA). The protein samples were added to sample buffer (2% SDS, 60mM Tris pH 6.8, 5% mercaptoethanol and 0.01% bromophenol blue) and subjected to electrophoresis on an SDS-PAGE system, 10% polyacrylamide gel (1.5M Tris-HCL, 10% SDS, 30% bis-acrylamide, 10% ammonium persulfate and TEMED). After electrophoresis, the proteins were transferred to nitrocellulose membranes (Bio-Rad, CA, USA) in a *semi-dry* transfer apparatus (*Semi-dry Transfer*, Bio-Rad, CA, USA). The membranes were incubated in blocking solution (SuperBlock T20(TBS) Blocking Buffer, Thermo scientific, USA) for 1 hour at room temperature and then washed in TBST (50mM Tris buffer, pH8.0, 100mM NaCl, 1% Tween 20) for 30 minutes and incubated with the primary antibody against the proteins of interest: Collagen type I (sc8784, dilution 1:1000, Santa Cruz, CA, USA); Collagen type III (sc28888, dilution 1:1000, Santa Cruz, CA, USA); FAK (ab40794, dilution 1:1000, Abcam Inc, MA, USA), pFAK (ab4803, dilution 1:1000, Abcam Inc, MA,

USA), Beta Actin (ab16039, dilution 1:1000, Abcam Inc, MA, USA).All the antibodies were incubated *overnight* at 4°C. Subsequently, the membranes were washed again with TBST and incubated in a solution containing peroxidase-conjugated secondary antibody (HRP goat *anti-rabbit* polyclonal- sc2004 or HRP *rabbit* anti-mouse, sc358923, dilution 1:20000, Santa Cruz, CA, USA) at room temperature for 1 hour. Finally, the membranes were washed with TBST and exposed to the detection system using the Super Signal chemiluminescent reagent (Pierce Rockford, IL, USA) and analyzed on a gel documenter (GBOX, Syngene, USA). The expression of the protein of interest was compared by gel densitometry using the "*GeneTools*" program (Syngene, USA), normalized by the control (control=1).

3.12 - Nitrite quantification - Griess reaction

The detection method was based on the reaction of nitrite with Griess reagent, producing a colorimetric reaction detected by absorbance at a wavelength of 595nm. The nitrate present in the sample was reduced to nitrite using the enzymes nitrate reductase and NADPH. The nitrite concentration was divided by the amount of protein present in the samples. For the Griess reaction, 100µl of working solution was added (solution A: 1% sulphanilamide in 5% phosphoric acid; and solution B: 0.1% naphthylethylenediamine in distilled water; mix equal parts of solutions A and B). After 10 minutes of incubation at room temperature, a reading was taken at a wavelength of 595nm on a SpectraMax^{TM} Microplate Reader (Molecular devises, Minnesota, USA).

3.13 - Fibroblast culture

Under sterile conditions, NIH-3T3 fibroblasts were thawed in a 37°C water bath and transferred to a 15 mL conical tube. 10 mL of DMEM culture medium was added and centrifuged at 1,000 rpm for 5 minutes to remove the DMSO from the freezing medium. The supernatant was discarded and the *pellet* was resuspended in 10 mL of DMEM culture medium supplemented with 10% fetal bovine serum, 1% antibiotic and antimycotic solution (penicillin 10,000 U, streptomycin 10,000 µg and 25 µg of amphotericin B) (GIBCO - Invitrogen, NY, USA). The cells were then plated in culture bottles using the same medium. The bottles were incubated at 37°C in an incubator with 5% CO_2 tension.

After reaching 80% confluence, the monolayer was resuspended in 0.25% trypsin solution (GIBCO - Invitrogen, NY, USA), incubated at 37°C for 5 minutes, followed by stopping the reaction by adding complete DMEM. The volume of the culture bottle was transferred to a conical tube and centrifuged at 1,000 rpm for 10 minutes, the supernatant was discarded, the *pellet* was resuspended with DMEM culture medium and plated again, representing the second passage. To carry out the experiments, $1x10^6$ cells/mL were plated in 6-well plates with 1 mL of DMEM medium.

3.13.1 - Stimulation of fibroblasts with LPS and hypertonic solution

The cells were resuspended at a concentration of $1x10^6$/mL and distributed in 6-well cell culture plates. The cells were separated into 4 groups:

- **Control group:**

The cells were maintained in DMEM culture medium without the addition of any other substance.

- **LPS group:**

After 24 hours of plating, the DMEM culture medium was replaced with DMEM containing *Escherichia coli* LPS (026:B6 Sigma, MO, USA) at a concentration of 1µg/mL.

- **LPS + HYPER group:**

After 24 hours of plating, the DMEM culture medium was replaced with DMEM containing *Escherichia coli* LPS (026:B6 Sigma, MO, USA) at a concentration of 1µg/mL. Four hours after exposing the cells to LPS, the medium was changed back to DMEM containing hypertonic solution with an osmolarity of 450 mOsm.

- **HIPER Group:**

After 24 hours of plating, the DMEM culture medium was replaced with DMEM containing hypertonic solution with an osmolarity of 450 mOsm. This group was not previously stimulated with LPS.

After 24 hours of exposure, cell extracts from all groups were collected and stored in a -80°C freezer for subsequent protein extraction and quantification of FAK and pFAK.

3.14 - Statistical analysis

Data is presented as mean±standard error of the mean. An analysis of variance (ANOVA) with Tukey's post-test was used for statistical analysis of the comparison of means, with groups obtaining $p<0.05$ being considered significant differences. The *GraphPad Prisma* - Version 5 program (*GraphPad Software Incorporation*) was used for data analysis. The Log rank test was used to analyze the survival curve.

RESULTS

4. Results

4.1 - Results of treated animals 15 minutes after LPS injection 4.1.1 - Mortality curve

The data obtained shows a higher mortality rate in the animals injected with LPS and those treated with normal saline after 15 minutes. After 48 hours, 20% of the animals in the LPS group died and 30% of the animals in the group injected with LPS and treated with normal saline. No animals died in the group treated with hypertonic solution during the period of analysis of animal mortality (figure 3).

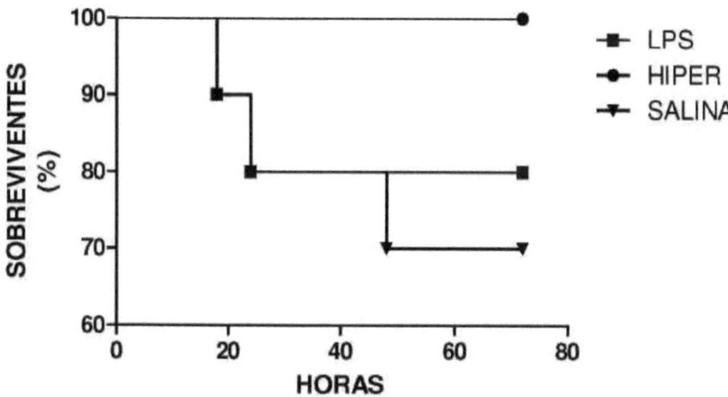

Figure 3. survival of Wistar rats separated into the LPS (injection of LPS 10mg/kg i.p.), Hyper (animals injected with LPS 10mg/kg i.p. treated with hypertonic saline NaCl 7.5% 4ml/kg i.v. 15 minutes after LPS) and Saline (animals injected with LPS 10mg/kg i.p. treated with saline solution NaCl 0.9% 34ml/kg i.v. 15 minutes after LPS) Survival was assessed every 12 hours for 72 hours. The results are expressed as percentage survival and the data presented are from 10 animals per group.

3.14.1 - Pulmonary edema

Pulmonary edema was assessed by determining the percentage of water in the organ. Figure 4 shows that there was a significant increase in the percentage of water in the tissue of the LPS and Saline groups when compared to the control group ($p<0.05$). The animals treated with hypertonic solution showed no significant increase in edema.

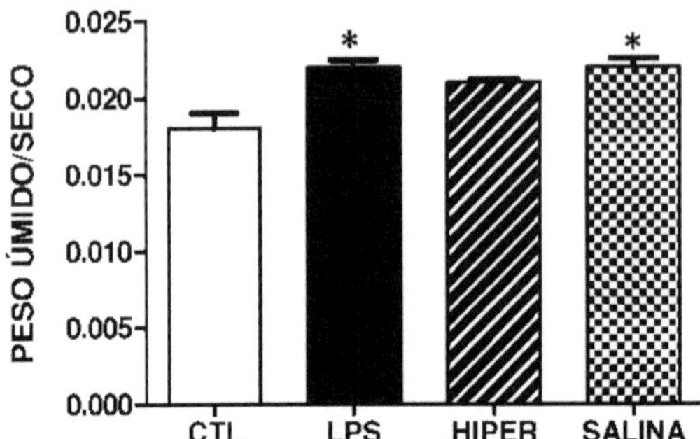

Figure 4: Percentage of water present in the lung tissue (ratio between wet and dry weight) of Wistar rats CTL (without any insult or treatment), LPS (injection of LPS 10mg/kg i.p.), Hyper (animals injected with LPS 10mg/kg i.p. treated with hypertonic solution NaCl 7.5% 4ml/kg i.v. 15 minutes after LPS) and Saline (animals injected with LPS 10mg/kg i.p. treated with saline solution NaCl 0.9% 34ml/kg i.v. 15 minutes after LPS) sacrificed 24 hours after treatment. Values expressed as mean±SEM and n=10 animals. $^{*}p<0.05$ vs. CTL.

3.14.2 - Production of Inflammatory Mediators

During endotoxemia, immune system cells are activated and inflammatory mediators are released, resulting in systemic inflammation. Thus, we evaluated whether treatment with hypertonic solution or saline solution would be able to inhibit the release of the pro-inflammatory cytokine TNF-α and the anti-inflammatory cytokine IL-10 in the lungs of endotoxemic animals.

We observed no significant differences between the groups with regard to the production of TNF-α and IL-10 within 24 hours.

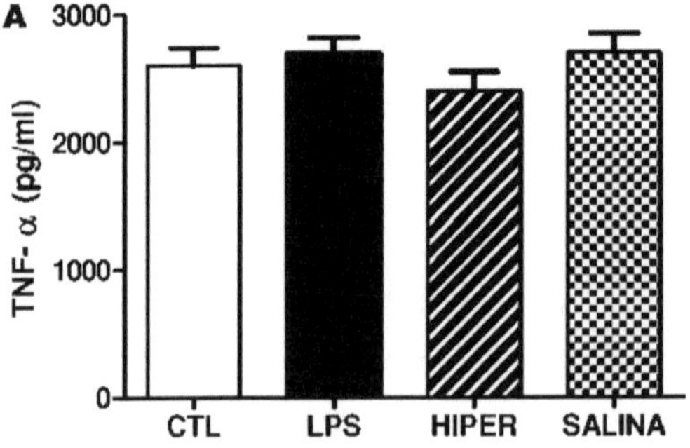

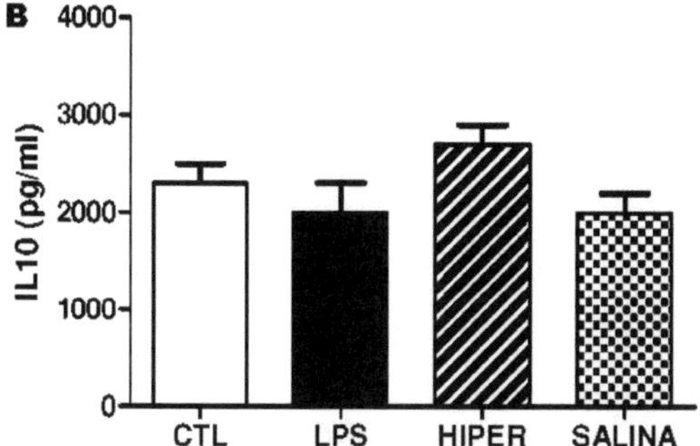

Figure 5 - Concentrations of TNF-α (A) and IL-10 (B) determined by ELISA in the lung tissue of Wistar rats CTL (without any insult or treatment), LPS (injection of LPS 10mg/kg i.p.), Hiper (animals injected with LPS 10mg/kg i..p. treated with hypertonic solution NaCl 7.5% 4ml/kg i.v. 15 minutes after LPS) and Saline (animals injected with LPS 10mg/kg i.p. treated with saline solution NaCl 0.9% 34ml/kg i.v. 15 minutes after LPS) and evaluated after 24 hours. Values expressed as mean±SEM and n=10 animals.

3.14.3 - Gene Expression of Metalloproteinase 9 (MMP-9)

Imetaloproteinases are responsible for the degradation of the extracellular matrix. The expression of MMP-9 is associated with tissue destruction in various diseases, including acute lung injury.

Our results show that MMP-9 gene expression increased significantly in endotoxemic animals 24 hours after disease induction ($p<0.05$). We also observed an increase in MMP-9 expression in the animals treated with saline solution, maintaining the same pattern observed in the animals without any treatment, both being significantly different from the control group ($p<0.05$).

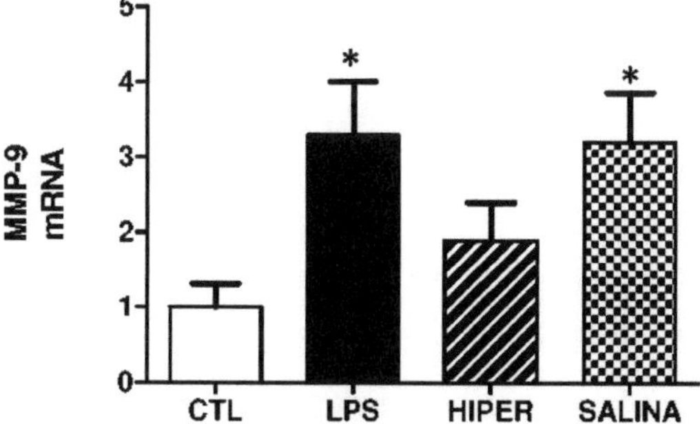

Figura 6. Gene expression in the lung of MMP-9 determined by real-time PCR of Wistar CTL rats (without any insult or treatment), LPS (injection of LPS 10mg/kg i.p), Hyper

(animals injected with LPS 10mg/kg i.p. treated with hypertonic solution NaCl 7.5% 4ml/kg i.v. 15 minutes after LPS) and Saline (animals injected with LPS 10mg/kg i.p. treated with saline solution NaCl 0.9% 34ml/kg i.v. 15 minutes after LPS) and evaluated after 24 hours. Values expressed as mean±SEM and n=10 animals. * $p<0.05$ vs Control.

4.1.5 - Metalloproteinase 9 (MMP 9) activity

We observed that the animals that received LPS injections tended to show an increase in MMP-9 activity, but when these animals were treated with saline, there was a significant increase in MMP-9 activity compared to all the other groups ($p<0.05$).

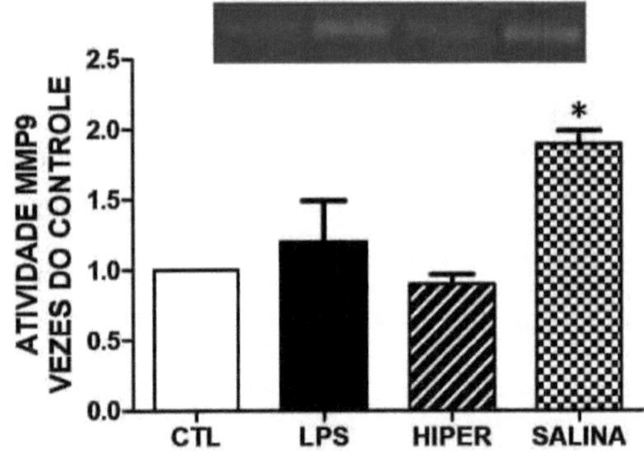

Figura 7. MMP-9 activity determined by zymography of Wistar rats CTL (without any insult or treatment), LPS (injection of LPS 10mg/kg i.p.), Hyper (animals injected with LPS 10mg/kg i.p. treated with hypertonic solution NaCl 7.5% 4ml/kg i.v. 15 minutes after LPS) and Saline (animals injected with LPS 10mg/kg i.p. treated with saline solution NaCl 0.9% 34ml/kg i.v. 15 minutes after LPS) and evaluated after 24 hours. Values expressed in times of the control (control=1) and n=3 animals. *$p<0.05$ vs other groups.

4.1.6 - Protein Expression of Type I and Type III Collagen

Increased deposition of type I collagen is related to greater resistance in lung tissue. Type III collagen has the characteristic of elastic fibers and is present in large quantities in the lungs. We therefore measured the protein expression of type I and type III collagen in order to see whether treatment with hypertonic saline prevented an imbalance in the deposition of these collagens in the lungs of endotoxemic animals.

We observed that the animals induced to endotoxemia showed a significant increase in the amount of type I collagen in the lung when compared to the CTL animals and the animals that received volume replacement ($p<0.05$). The animals in the saline group showed an increase in collagen deposition when compared to the animals treated with hypertonic saline and the CTL animals (*p<0.05*).

With regard to the deposition of type III collagen, which gives elasticity to lung tissue, we observed that treatment with hypertonic saline showed a tendency to prevent a decrease in this collagen in the lung tissue; this was different from what happened with the untreated animals or those treated with saline. However, there was no significant difference between the groups.

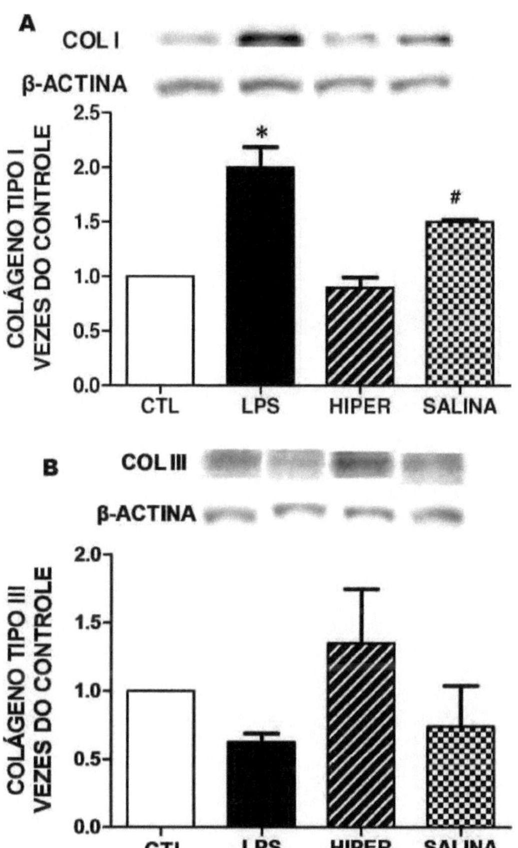

Figure 8. Protein expression in the lung of type I (A) and type III (B) collagens determined by Western Blot of Wistar rats CTL (without any insult or treatment), LPS (injection of LPS 10mg/kg i.p), Hiper (animals injected with LPS 10mg/kg i..p. treated with hypertonic NaCl 7.5% 4ml/kg i.v. 15 minutes after LPS) and Saline (animals injected with LPS 10mg/kg i.p. treated with saline NaCl 0.9% 34ml/kg i.v. 15 minutes after LPS) evaluated after 24 hours.

Values expressed in times of the control (control=1) and n=3 animals. *$p<0.05$ vs. other groups; # $p<0.05$ vs. CTL and Hyper.

4.1.7 - Lung function

Based on the results in which we observed that treatment with hypertonic solution was able to prevent the imbalance between the deposition of type I and type III collagens in the lung tissue of endotoxemic rats, we assessed the respiratory mechanics of these animals in order to see if this would improve their respiratory function. The graphs show that the animals in the LPS group and the animals treated with saline, unlike the animals treated with hypertonic, showed an increase in pulmonary resistance ($p<0.05$) (Figure 9A).

With regard to elastance, we observed a significant increase in the animals treated with saline when compared to the control group ($p<0.05$) (Figure 9B).

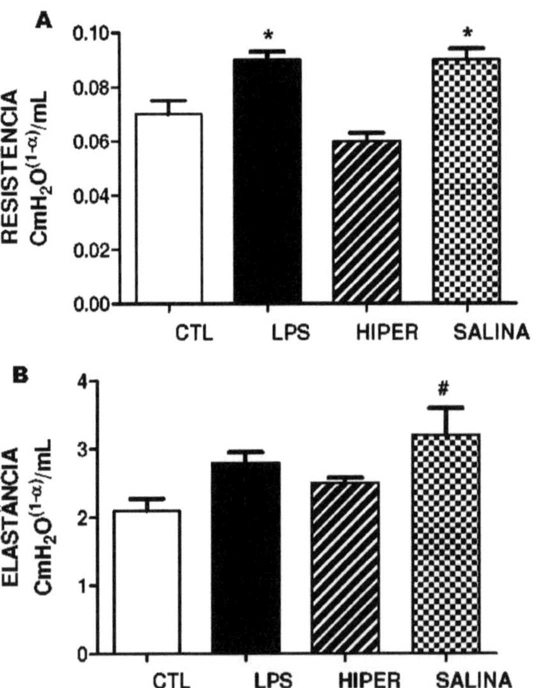

Figure 9. Evaluation of the resistance (A) and elastance (B) of the lung tissue of Wistar CTL rats (without any insult or treatment), LPS (injection of LPS 10mg/kg i.p.), Hyper (animals injected with LPS 10mg/kg i.p. treated with hypertonic solution NaCl 7.5% 4ml/kg i.v. 15 minutes after LPS) and Saline (animals injected with LPS 10mg/kg i.p. treated with saline solution NaCl 0.9% 34ml/kg i.v. 15 minutes after LPS), evaluated 24 hours after treatment.

Values expressed as mean±SEM and n=10 animals. *$p<0.05$ vs. Control and HYPER, # $p<0.05$ vs. Control.

4.1.8 - Activating FAK

Activation of focal adhesion kinase (FAK) has been linked to the onset of the remodeling mechanism in various models of lung injury. In order to see if the treatment of endotoxemic animals with saline or hypertonic solution is capable of modulating this pathway, we measured the expression of FAK in the lung tissue of these animals.

We observed that FAK activity increased significantly in the animals injected with LPS and in the animals treated with saline solution, when compared to the CTL and hypertonic solution-treated groups ($p<0.05$) 24 hours after treatment (figure 10).

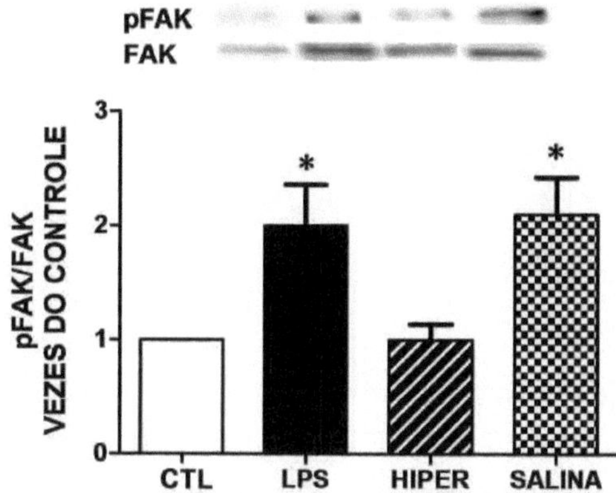

Figura 10. FAK activation in the lung determined by Western Blot of Wistar rats CTL (without any insult or treatment), LPS (injection of LPS 10mg/kg i.p.), Hyper (animals injected with LPS 10mg/kg i.p. treated with hypertonic NaCl 7.5% 4ml/kg i.v. 15 minutes after LPS) and Saline (animals injected with LPS 10mg/kg i.p. treated with saline NaCl 0.9% 34ml/kg i.v. 15 minutes after LPS) and evaluated after 24 hours. Values expressed in times of the control (control=1) and n=3 animals. *$p<0.05$ vs CTL and Hyper.

4.1.9 - Action of hypertonic solution on the FAK pathway

Based on the results presented above, we observed that treatment with hypertonic saline prevented the deposition of collagen in the lung, and that this process may be related to the inhibition of focal adhesion kinase (FAK). We therefore decided to explore the pathways involved in this process in order to elucidate the mechanism of action of hypertonic saline on lung remodeling in endotoxemic rats.

Our first hypothesis was that the increase in osmolarity promoted by the injection of hypertonic solution would alter the cytoskeleton of the cells, leading to inhibition of FAK and, consequently, a decrease in collagen production.

We observed that the cells treated with LPS and those kept in culture medium with hypertonic solution showed an increase in FAK expression when compared to the CTL group (*p<0.05*) (figure 11). These results suggest that the mechanism of action of hypertonic solution through inhibition of FAK does not occur in response to changes in the cytoskeleton as a result of increased osmolarity.

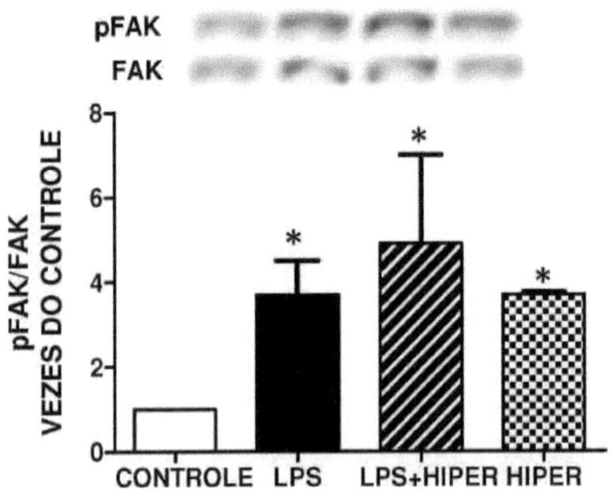

Figura 11. FAK activity in cell culture of fibroblasts separated into control groups (kept in DMEM culture medium), LPS (stimulated with 10µg/mL LPS), LPS + Hyper (4 hours after stimulation with LPS, the medium was changed to hypertonic 450 mOsm medium), Hyper (cells kept in hypertonic 450 mOsm medium). 24 hours after exposure, the cells were collected and the proteins extracted for Western Blotting. Values expressed in times of the control (control=1) of 2 independent experiments n=3 per experiment. *$p<0.05$ vs. Control.

4.1.10 - Action of hypertonic solution on nitric oxide synthesis

Some authors have shown that the expression of nitric oxide in the lung is closely related to the deposition of collagen in the tissue and that this mechanism involves the activation of FAK. In order to see whether treatment with hypertonic saline would decrease NO production, leading to FAK inactivation and a consequent decrease in collagen deposition, we measured iNOS expression in the lung tissue and the amount of nitrite, a NO by-product, in the animals' plasma.

The graphs show that the expression of iNOS in the tissue of the endotoxemic animals that received no treatment and the animals treated with saline was increased when compared to the CTL and HIPER groups (p<0.05) (Figure 12A). With regard to nitrite, there was an increase in its production in the LPS and Saline groups when compared to the CTL group (*p*<0.05) (Figure 12B).

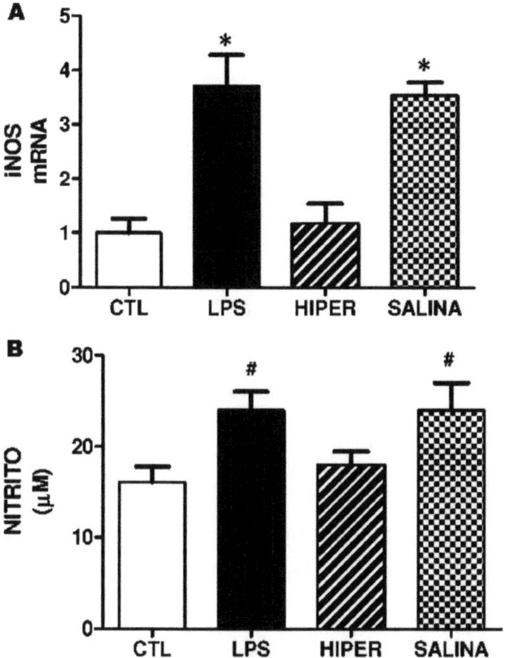

Figure 12. Gene expression in the lung of iNOS (A) determined by real-time PCR and quantification of nitrite by the Griess method in the plasma (B) of Wistar rats CTL (without any insult or treatment), LPS (injection of LPS 10mg/kg i.p), Hiper (animals injected with LPS 10mg/kg i.p. treated with hypertonic NaCl 7.5% 4ml/kg i.v. 15 minutes after LPS) and Saline (animals injected with LPS 10mg/kg i.p. treated with saline NaCl 0.9% 34ml/kg i.v. 15 minutes after LPS) and evaluated 24 hours after treatment. Values expressed as mean±EPM and n=10 animals. *p<0.05 vs CTL and Hyper; # p<0.05 vs. CTL.

4.2 - Results of animals treated 1.5 hours after LPS injection

In order to bring our results closer to clinical practice, we evaluated the effect of late treatment (1.5 hours after inducing endotoxemia) with hypertonic saline and saline solution on the lungs of animals exposed to LPS, 24 hours after treatment.

4.2.1 - Mortality Curve

In order to see whether late treatment (1.5 hours after inducing endotoxemia) would continue to be effective, we performed a mortality curve on the endotoxemic and late-treated animals. The data show that, unlike what we observed in the early treatment of endotoxemia, the animals treated with saline and hypertonic solution showed mortality close to that of the untreated animals.

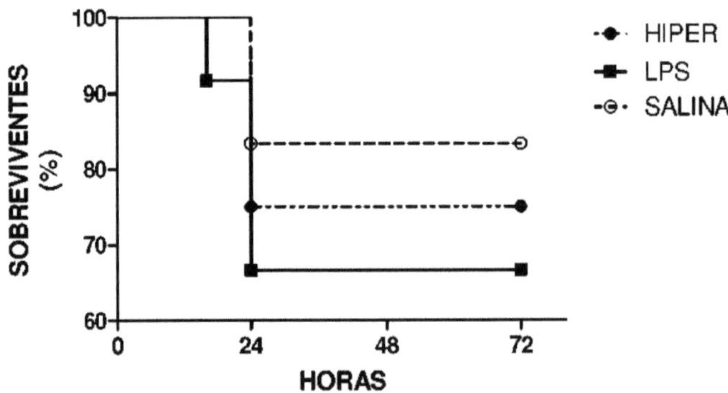

Figure 13. Survival of Wistar rats separated into the LPS (injection of LPS 10mg/kg i.p.), Hyper (animals injected with LPS 10mg/kg i.p. treated with hypertonic solution NaCl 7.5% 4ml/kg i.v.) and Saline (animals injected with LPS 10mg/kg i.p. treated with hypertonic solution NaCl 0.9% 34ml/kg i.v.) groups. 1.5 hours after LPS) and Saline (animals injected with LPS 10mg/kg i.p. treated with saline solution NaCl 0.9% 34ml/kg i.v. 1.5 hours after LPS) Survival was assessed every 12 hours for 72 hours. The results are expressed as percentage survival and the data presented are from 12 animals per group.

4.2.2 - Pulmonary edema

We observed that the animals treated 1.5 hours after LPS injection and sacrificed 24 hours after treatment showed a tendency to reduce the percentage of water. This improvement, however, was not significant.

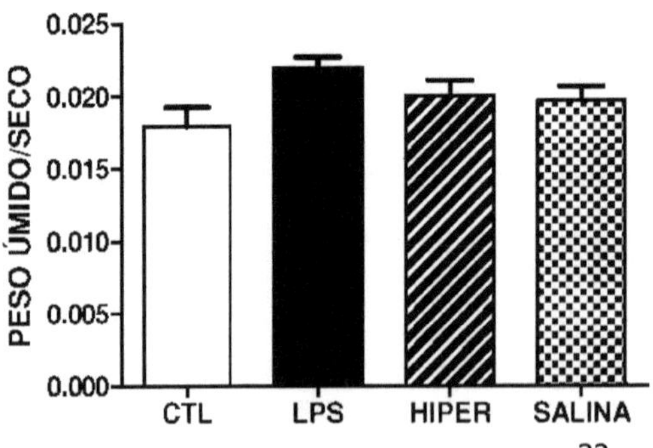

Figure 14. Percentage of water present in the lung tissue (ratio between wet and dry weight) of Wistar rats CTL (without any insult or treatment), LPS (injection of LPS 10mg⁄kg i.p), Hiper (animals injected with LPS 10mg⁄kg i.p. treated with hypertonic solution NaCl 7.5% 4ml⁄kg i.v. 1.5 hours after LPS) and Saline (animals injected with LPS 10mg⁄kg i.p. treated with saline solution NaCl 0.9% 34ml/kg i.v. 1.5 hours after LPS) sacrificed 24 hours after treatment. Values expressed as mean±SEM and n=10 animals.

4.2.3 - Production of Inflammatory Mediators

In order to see whether late treatment could alter the production of the pro-inflammatory cytokine TNF-α and the anti-inflammatory cytokine IL-10, we measured their expression in the lung tissue of endotoxemic and treated animals.

Our results show that both treatments were responsible for worsening the inflammatory parameters of lung tissue, increasing the amount of TNF-α when compared to CTL and LPS animals ($p<0.05$), and decreasing IL-10 when compared to the same groups ($p<0.05$).

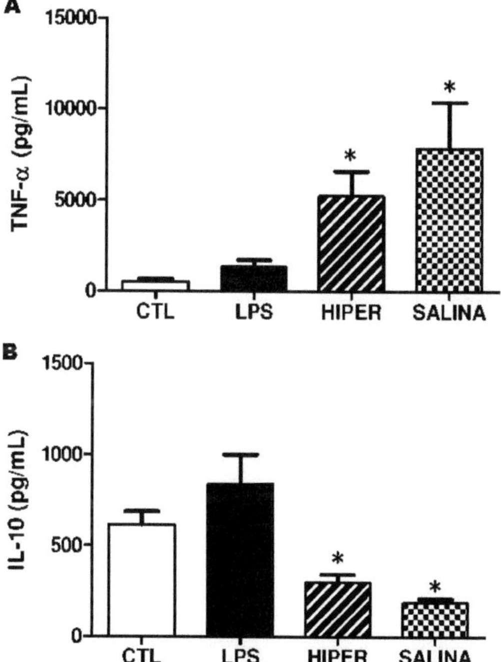

Figure 15. Concentrations of TNF-α (A) and IL-10 (B) determined by ELISA in the lung tissue of Wistar rats CTL (without any insult or treatment), LPS (injection of LPS 10mg⁄kg i.p), Hyper (animals injected with LPS 10mg⁄kg i.p. treated with hypertonic solution NaCl

7.5% 4ml/kg i.v. 1.5 hours after LPS) and Saline (animals injected with LPS 10mg/kg i.p. treated with saline solution NaCl 0.9% 34ml/kg i.v. 1.5 hours after LPS) and evaluated after 24 hours. Values expressed as mean±SEM and n=10 animals. *$p<0.05$ vs. CTL and LPS.

4.2.4 - Gene Expression of Metalloproteinase 9 (MMP-9)

In order to observe the action of late treatment with saline and hypertonic solution on tissue remodeling, we measured the gene expression of MMP-9 in lung tissue.

Our results show that MMP-9 gene expression increased significantly in animals treated with saline and hypertonic solution 1.5 hours after endotoxemia induction when compared to the CTL and LPS groups ($p<0.05$).

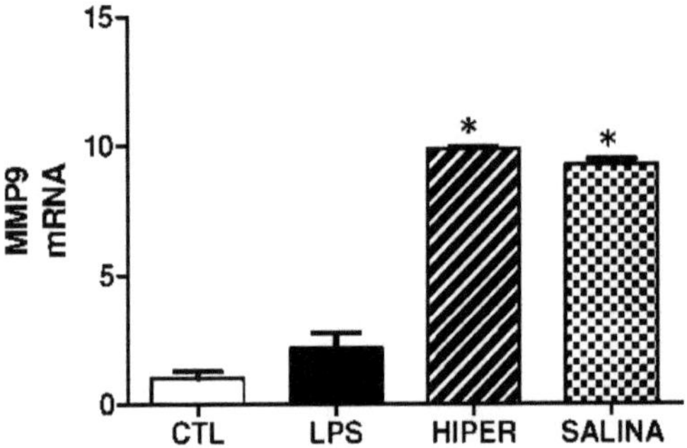

Figure 16. MMP-9 gene expression in the lung determined by real-time PCR of Wistar rats CTL (without any insult or treatment), LPS (injection of LPS 10mg/kg i.p.), Hiper (animals injected with LPS 10mg/kg i.p. treated with hypertonic solution NaCl 7.5% 4ml/kg i.v. 1.5 hours after LPS) and Salina (animals injected with LPS 10mg/kg i.p.). treated with hypertonic solution NaCl 7.5% 4ml/kg i.v. 1.5 hours after LPS) and Saline (animals injected with LPS 10mg/kg i.p. treated with saline solution NaCl 0.9% 34ml/kg i.v. 1.5 hours after LPS) and evaluated 24 hours after treatment. Values expressed as mean±SEM and n=10 animals. * $p<0.05$ vs CTL and LPS.

4.2.5 - Metalloproteinase 9 (MMP 9) activity

Following the profile observed in the gene expression of MMP-9, we observed that the activity of MMP-9 increased in the animals treated with saline and hypertonic saline 1.5 hours after the induction of endotoxemia, but this difference was not significant in relation to the other groups.

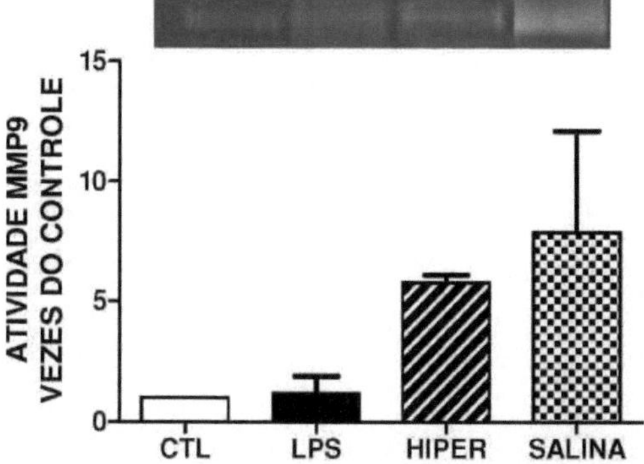

Figure 17. MMP-9 activity determined by zymography of Wistar CTL rats (without any insult or treatment), LPS (injection of LPS 10mg/kg i.p.), Hyper (animals injected with LPS 10mg/kg i.p. treated with hypertonic NaCl 7.5% 4ml/kg i.v. 1.5 hours after LPS) and Saline (animals injected with LPS 10mg/kg i.p. treated with saline NaCl 0.9% 34ml/kg i.v. 1.5 hours after LPS) and evaluated after 24 hours. Values expressed in times of the control (control=1) and n=3 animals.

4.2.6 - Protein Expression of Type I and Type III Collagen

Our previous results showed that treatment with hypertonic saline at an early stage was able to decrease the protein expression of type I collagen and prevent a decrease in type III collagen 24 hours after treatment. Thus, we evaluated whether treatment with hypertonic solution would also be effective in balancing the deposition of type I and type III collagen in the lung tissue of animals treated 1.5 hours after the induction of endotoxemia.

Our results showed that contrary to what was observed in the animals treated at during the early stages of the disease, the deposition of type I collagen was not reduced compared to the animals that were not treated. Treatment with hypertonic solution was also unable to prevent a decrease in type III collagen in the lung tissue.

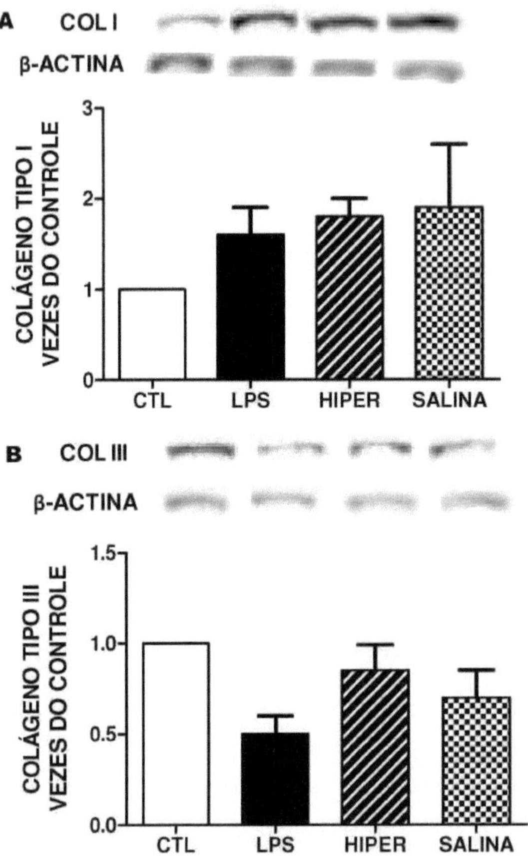

Figure 18. Protein expression in the lung of type I collagen (A) and type III collagen (B) determined by Western Blot of Wistar rats CTL (without any insult or treatment), LPS (injection of LPS 10mg/kg i.p), Hyper (animals injected with LPS 10mg/kg i.p. treated with hypertonic NaCl 7.5% 4ml/kg i.v. 1.5 hours after LPS) and Saline (animals injected with LPS 10mg/kg i.p. treated with saline NaCl 0.9% 34ml/kg i.v. 1.5 hours after LPS). Assessed 24 hours after treatment. Values expressed in times of the control (control=1) and n=3 animals.

4.2.7 - Lung function

In order to see whether the late treatment of endotoxemic animals with saline solution or hypertonic solution leads to an improvement in lung mechanics 24 hours after treatment, we measured the resistance and elastance of the tissue.

The graphs show that both treatments, despite showing a tendency to increase resistance and elastance, did not significantly alter lung mechanics parameters.

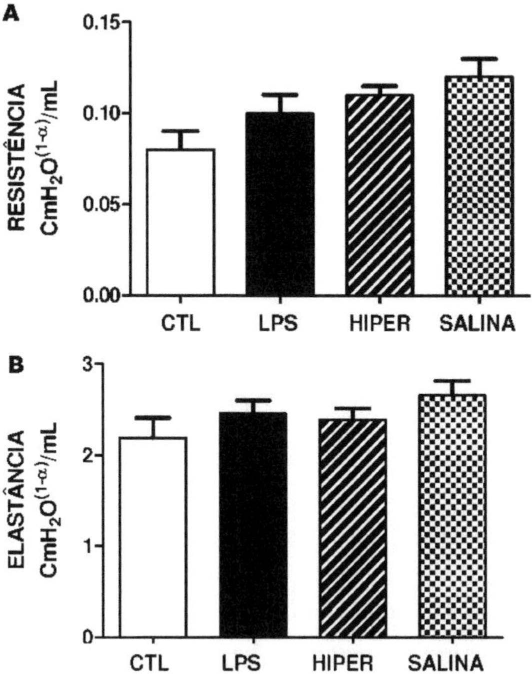

Figure 19. Pulmonary function assessment (tissue resistance (A) and elastance (B)) of Wistar CTL rats (without any insult or treatment), LPS (injection of LPS 10mg/kg i.p.), Hyper (animals injected with LPS 10mg/kg i.p. treated with hypertonic solution NaCl 7.5% 4ml/kg i.v. 1.5 hours after LPS) and Saline (animals injected with LPS 10mg/kg i.p. treated with saline solution NaCl 0.9% 34ml/kg i.v. 1.5 hours after LPS) and evaluated 24 hours after treatment. Values expressed as mean±SEM and n=10 animals.

4.2.8 - Activating FAK

As we have previously shown, collagen deposition in lung tissue is related to FAK activation. Our results showed that late treatment with hypertonic solution did not prevent tissue remodeling through collagen deposition, so we evaluated FAK activity in order to see if its activation was related to collagen deposition.

We observed that FAK activity was increased in the lung tissue of animals treated with saline and hypertonic solution, in line with the results observed in relation to collagen deposition.

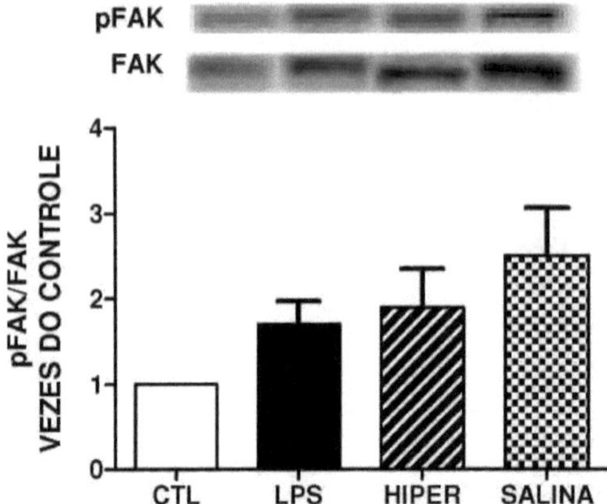

Figura 20. FAK activation in the lung determined by Western Blot of Wistar rats CTL (without any insult or treatment), LPS (injection of LPS 10mg/kg i.p.), Hyper (animals injected with LPS 10mg/kg i.p. treated with hypertonic NaCl 7.5% 4ml/kg i.v. 1.5 hours after LPS) and Saline (animals injected with LPS 10mg/kg i.p. treated with saline solution NaCl 0.9% 34ml/kg i.v. 1.5 hours after LPS) and evaluated after 24 hours. Values expressed in times of the control (control=1) and n=3 animals.

4.2.9 - Action of late treatment with hypertonic solution on nitric oxide synthesis

Early treatment of endotoxemic rats with hypertonic saline showed a decrease in the expression of iNOS and nitrite 24 hours after treatment. Thus, we evaluated whether late treatment with hypertonic saline or saline also modulated these mediators

We observed that both saline and hypertonic saline treatments increased iNOS expression when compared to the CTL and LPS groups ($p<0.05$) (figure 21A). The group treated with hypertonic solution also showed a significantly greater increase in iNOS expression than the animals treated with saline solution (.05). As for nitrite (figure 21B), we observed that the treatments did not reduce its production in the plasma of the endotoxemic animals.

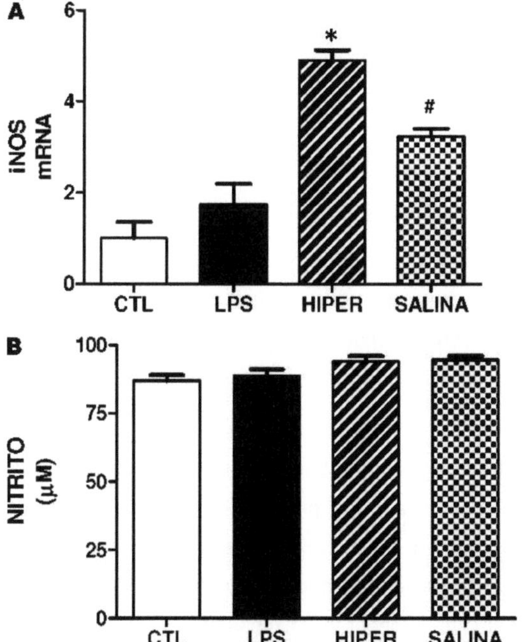

Figura 21. Gene expression of iNOS in the lung (A) determined by real-time PCR and quantification of nitrite by the Griess method in the plasma (B) of Wistar rats CTL (without any insult or treatment), LPS (injection of LPS 10mg/kg i.p.), Hiper (animals injected with LPS 10mg/kg i.p. treated with hypertonic solution NaCl 7.5% 4ml/kg i.v. 1.5 hours after LPS) and Saline (animals injected with LPS 10mg/kg i.p. treated with saline solution NaCl 0.9% 34ml/kg i.v. 1.5 hours after LPS) and evaluated 24 hours after treatment. Values expressed as mean±SEM and n=10 animals. *$p<0.05$ vs. other groups; # $p<0.05$ vs. CTL.

DISCUSSION

5. Discussion

Sepsis is a serious disease characterized by a systemic inflammatory response and is one of the leading causes of death in non-coronary ICUs (98).

Despite great advances in understanding the pathogenesis of sepsis, the mortality rate in patients with the disease remains high. The lung is among the first organs to be affected during multiple organ failure caused by worsening sepsis. In this context, acute respiratory distress syndrome (ARDS) is among the leading causes of death in septic patients admitted to intensive care units (27, 48, 49, 99).

Early fluid resuscitation is an essential strategy in the treatment of septic shock. Early fluid resuscitation can considerably improve the patient's prognosis, reducing mortality. Prospective studies in patients with ARDS have associated the strategy of reduced volume administration with improved oxygenation and a reduction in the number of days patients spend on mechanical ventilation. Other studies suggest that excessive fluid infusion leads to fluid retention in the interstitial space, aggravating lung damage. Thus, the best course of action for patients with ARDS resulting from sepsis remains a major challenge for doctors (4, 100).

Volume resuscitation with hypertonic saline (7.5% NaCl) has been shown to be effective in recovering plasma volume and blood pressure due to the mobilization of fluids from the intracellular space to extracellular compartments. Some studies show that hypertonicity can also act on the immune system by activating genes, regulating protein expression, activating kinases involved in cell signaling and regulating cytokines (101, 102).

In the lung, the use of hypertonic solution as a therapy promotes a reduction in lung damage after septic and hemorrhagic shock. Studies have shown that hypertonic solution reduces neutrophil accumulation and histopathological damage in the lung (80, 103).

5.2 - Effects of early treatment with hypertonic solution

The exacerbated inflammatory response observed in patients with sepsis causes cell damage which often leads to the patient's death (34). In this context, our results showed that the animals that received treatment with hypertonic solution did not die, unlike the animals that were injected with LPS and did not receive treatment and the animals that were treated with saline solution. This result suggests that early treatment with hypertonic solution is more effective in controlling the effects of the disease, preventing mortality in these animals.

Our results are in line with those observed by other authors who showed that treating septic patients with hypertonic solution reduced the incidence of complications and, consequently, their mortality (104, 105). These effects may be related to a reduction in the inflammatory response, as well as a reduction in tissue damage.

One of the characteristics of acute lung injury is the appearance of pulmonary edema. The relative organ weight ratio expresses the accumulation of fluid in the organs and, although it is not a very sensitive method, it is simple and reliable to obtain. Volume replacement with the use of large volumes, as well as severe inflammatory processes, is associated with tissue edema (106). We observed that the induction of endotoxemia and treatment with saline solution increased pulmonary edema in the animals when compared to the control group 24 hours after LPS injection, showing that endotoxemia and volume replacement with saline solution increase the amount of extravascular pulmonary fluid, possibly due to the large amount of fluid administered.

The increase in lung weight indicates a greater accumulation of fluids in this organ, which can lead to functional alterations, especially in gas exchange, resulting in functional impairment (40). Thus, we can see that early treatment with smaller volumes of hypertonic solution can bring important benefits in terms of pulmonary impairment in ARDS patients. Some studies have reported that the peak of pulmonary edema in endotoxemic animals occurs 6 hours after LPS injection and gradually resolves (40). This may be related to our results, suggesting that the effects of volume replacement in these animals could be more evident in earlier periods than those studied in this study. Endotoxemia is characterized by causing an early and intense inflammatory response in the lung. Studies show that 2 hours after the induction of endotoxemia, inflammatory cell infiltration and thickening of the alveolar septum are observed, peaking at 24 hours (40).

It is known that endotoxemia can directly activate macrophages, endothelial cells and the complement system, triggering the release of various pro-inflammatory mediators such as TNF-α, interleukins IL-1β and IL-6, nitric oxide, among others, as well as the release of anti-inflammatory proteins such as IL-10, IL-4 and TGF-β (38). The main objective of our study was to analyze the action of treatment with hypertonic solution on the tissue remodeling process. For this reason, we decided to analyze the pro-inflammatory cytokine TNF-α and the anti-inflammatory cytokine IL-10 in order to see if the inflammatory process was also being modulated by the treatment.

TNF-α is mainly produced by macrophages and T cells after stimulation by LPS and is considered a potent activator of macrophages, neutrophils and endothelial cells. High concentrations of TNF-α have been linked to mortality in experimental sepsis studies (64). IL-10 is a potent anti-inflammatory cytokine responsible for decreasing the production of pro-inflammatory mediators, inhibiting the proliferation of T-cells, as well as protecting animals in LPS endotoxemia models (38, 107).

Our results showed no differences between the groups in relation to the production of TNF-α and IL-10, 24 hours after induction of the disease. However, it was possible to observe a tendency for the group treated with hypertonic to favorably modulate the levels of these cytokines by decreasing TNF-α and increasing IL-10. Studies show that the expression of TNF-α and IL-10 show an early response, a few hours after the induction of endotoxemia (40), so possibly in earlier periods we could observe greater differences between the treatments. Rojas et al (40) showed that these cytokines show early peaks, occurring 2 hours after induction of the disease and returning to baseline values after 24 hours. These results are in line with those observed in this study.

Alterations in the regulation of the enzymatic machinery involved in the degradation of ECM is a factor that contributes to various pathogeneses, including acute lung injury (61). These proteolytic enzymes include metalloproteinases (MMPs). MMPs are necessary for the degradation of ECM, but have been related to the modification of the immune system through the release of apoptotic proteins and cytokines. Among the metalloproteinases, MMP-9 plays an important role in tissue damage (108). Metalloproteinase 9 (MMP-9) is characterized by its ability to digest collagens, and its action has been related to various pathologies such as inflammation, neurodegeneration and lung damage (60). In order to see if the results observed in the animals treated with hypertonic saline were related to a reduction in lung damage, we measured their gene expression and MMP-9 activity.

We observed that the animals treated with hypertonic saline showed a decrease in gene expression and MMP-9 activity when compared to the animals treated with saline. Several studies have shown the important role that MMP-9 plays in the degradation of lung tissue and consequent damage to this tissue (109, 110). The action of MMP-9 could be responsible for the increase in collagen deposition in lung tissue, leading to fibrosis (109).

Studies have shown that patients with sepsis-induced ARDS have twice as much collagen in their lungs (50). This increase in collagen deposition may be related to the high mortality rates observed in ARDS patients as a result of progressive respiratory dysfunction (50). Among the various types of collagens, type I and III collagens are among the most important for lung tissue. Type I collagen is a thicker fiber and its main characteristic is increased tissue tension. Collagen III has thinner fibrils which, when aggregated, form fine fibers.

These fibers form the flexible reticular network of parenchymal organs such as the liver, pancreas and lung.

We observed that treatment with hypertonic saline prevented the expression of type I collagen in the lungs of the animals, unlike treatment with saline, which was not effective in regulating it. As for collagen III, we observed that treatment with hypertonic saline prevented its reduction, unlike what happened in the animals that received LPS and the animals that were treated with saline. In the lung, the increase in the deposition of type I collagen is related to an increase in pulmonary resistance, causing significant damage to respiratory function (111, 112). Some authors suggest that during ARDS, collagen III, which is more flexible, is replaced by collagen I, which is more rigid, which leads to a reduction in lung compliance and the patient may need mechanical ventilation (44, 113). Thus, treatment with hypertonic saline shows promise in controlling this imbalance and, consequently, pulmonary dysfunction.

Tissue repair involves the ability of fibroblasts to attach to the extracellular matrix through specialized structures called focal adhesions, resulting in cell migration and contraction of the ECM (114). The mechanism of adhesion to the ECM involves integrins, whose signals are transmitted by focal adhesion *kinase* (FAK). FAK expression is directly related to the migration of fibroblasts into lung tissue (115). An increase in its expression and activity contributes to the formation of fibrosis in the tissue (115).

Our results showed that the animals injected with LPS and those treated with saline had a significant increase in FAK activity, but when the animals were treated with hypertonic saline, the activity of this protein was inhibited. This inactivation may be related to the decrease in collagen deposition in the lung tissue of the hypertonic-treated animals. Our group recently published two studies showing that inactivation of FAK through the use of RNA interference decreased collagen deposition in the blood and lungs of endotoxemic rats, suggesting that this pathway could be an important therapeutic target in this disease (56, 116).

Other studies have linked the expression of FAK with the production of metalloproteinase 9, showing that the role of FAK in cell migration is related to the degradation of ECM through the action of metalloproteinases (117, 118). Thus, a possible explanation for the increase in MMP-9 expression and activity observed in our study could be the result of the increase in FAK expression in the endotoxemic animals and in the animals that received saline solution. Together, these results show that the decrease in collagen deposition observed in the animals that received hypertonic saline could be occurring through this pathway.

Based on the results in the literature and our own results, we decided to study the way in which the hypertonic solution was acting during this process.

Initially, we evaluated whether the increase in osmolarity was inhibiting FAK activation in fibroblasts. Our results showed that when fibroblasts are kept in a culture medium with hypertonic solution, there is an increase in FAK activation. Among the known functions of FAK, its action as a mediator of signals from the extracellular to the intracellular environment from integrins stands out. Its activation is related to mechanotransduction, resulting from the stress suffered by the cell (90). Thus, our results suggest that the inactivation of FAK by the hypertonic solution was not due to its direct action on the cell's cytoskeleton, and that its inhibition was the result of the action of other pathways involved in the tissue remodeling process.

Recent studies have shown that FAK activation can occur in response to neutrophil migration and that this process is dependent on nitric oxide (NO) (119-121). In order to see if the inactivation of FAK that occurred in the tissue of the animals that received hypertonics was related to the decrease in NO, we measured induced nitric oxide synthase (iNOS) in the lung tissue and nitrite, a by-product of NO, in the plasma. Our results showed that treatment with hypertonic solution inhibited both the expression of iNOS in the tissue and nitrite in the plasma of the animals.

In a recent study, it was observed that FAK activation could occur during the process of neutrophil infiltration into the tissue, through the activation of adhesion molecules (121). It is known that neutrophil accumulation in the lung occurs through the signaling of effector molecules such as free radicals, cytokines and nitric oxide (NO) (65, 69). NO synthesis differs in the amount and time of release depending on the type of NO synthase active. The induced form (iNOS) synthesizes NO in large quantities during inflammatory processes. This leads to increased neutrophil and macrophage activation (122). Although it was not possible to quantify neutrophil infiltration in our study, it is widely established in the literature that among the actions performed by hypertonic saline, the reduction in neutrophil infiltration in the tissue is widely established (73, 123). Thus, our results suggest that the decrease in collagen deposition in lung tissue through the inactivation of FAK observed in the animals treated with hypertonic saline is related to the decrease in NO and, consequently, to the possible decrease in neutrophil infiltration in the tissue. This result may also explain the decrease in the expression and activity of metalloproteinase 9 (MMP-9) observed in the tissue. Neutrophils are the main MMP-9 secreting cells, which are present in latent form in their granules. Thus, as neutrophil infiltration decreases, there is less release of MMP-9, which leads to a consequent reduction in tissue damage.

Among the characteristics of acute lung injury, we observed a fibroproliferative phase with collagen deposition and consequent loss of lung function (124). Through lung mechanics analyses, we observed that treatment with hypertonic saline decreased the resistance of the lung tissue of endotoxemic animals and saline was responsible for an increase in tissue elastance. These results are in line with

This is contrary to expectations, considering the decrease in collagen deposition observed in the animals treated with hypertonic solution. Several studies have shown that the increase in the deposition of collagen fibers in lung tissue is related to the changes observed in the resistance and elastance of lung tissue (109, 113, 125).

As a result, patients with ARDS have altered lung mechanics and do not respond normally to recruitment maneuvers (126).

It is known that a large proportion of septic patients who enter the ICU have reduced lung function, requiring mechanical ventilation. Several studies have shown that mechanical ventilation may be responsible for increased damage to lung tissue, leading to an increase in collagen deposition in the tissue (39, 127). Our results confirmed the therapeutic potential of hypertonic solution. We observed that treatment with hypertonic solution can avoid the need to use mechanical ventilation, reducing the incidence of pulmonary complications resulting from its use.

5.3 - Effects of delayed treatment with hypertonic solution

The great difficulty in reproducing the results found in animal models treated with hypertonic solution when applied to patients is related to the period during which the treatment is carried out.

The beneficial action of hypertonic solution when administered in the early stages of the disease is well-established, but several studies carried out with patients have not shown similar results.

Some authors suggest that the time of administration is more important than the type of fluid used (128, 129).

In order to see if the late treatment of endotoxemic animals would show different results to those observed in animals treated early in the induction of the disease, we analyzed the action of the hypertonic solution 1.5 hours after the induction of the disease. This is the period in which most of the inflammatory mediators show their maximum expression.

Our results showed that delayed treatment with hypertonic solution was unable to prevent mortality in endotoxemic animals, and was worse than treatment with saline solution. These results may explain the lack of positive results regarding the mortality of septic patients when treated with hypertonic solution. It is known that it is difficult to administer volume early in clinical practice.

In a study published by Gao et al. (130), which compared two strategies of volume administration in septic patients, one of which was early and the other late, it was observed that those patients treated early showed a great reduction in mortality when compared to those treated late. More recently, the prospective randomized study published by van Haren and collaborators (131), although it showed an improvement in the microcirculation of septic patients, did not show any benefits of hypertonic solution in altering the mortality rate of these patients.

As for pulmonary edema, as we observed with early treatment, there was no significant decrease in the percentage of water in the lungs of the animals in either treatment. The lack of difference may be related to the study period.

Some studies have shown that early treatment with hypertonic solution reduces damage to lung tissue, while late treatment significantly increases oxidative stress and the accumulation of polymorphonuclear neutrophils in the lung, aggravating lung tissue damage after sepsis (101, 132).

Our results showed that 1.5 hours after treatment of the endotoxemic animals, contrary to what occurred in the animals treated early, there was an increase in the expression and activity of MMP-9 in the lung tissue of the animals treated with hypertonic solution or saline solution. These results suggest that late treatments may increase tissue damage due to an increase in MMP-9 activity. This may be due to a greater accumulation of inflammatory cells in the tissue.

Inoue et al. (132) showed that late treatment with hypertonic solution of septic animals was responsible for an increase in neutrophil infiltration in the lung tissue, when compared to animals that received treatment 15 minutes after induction of the disease. Other studies have shown similar results, indicating that treatment with hypertonic solution can have opposite effects such as neutrophil activation or inhibition, depending on the period of administration, being ineffective when administered after neutrophil activation (133, 134). Therefore, these results suggest that late treatment of the disease could cause an increase in the infiltration of inflammatory cells in the lung tissue, which could increase tissue damage.

With regard to the deposition of collagens in lung tissue, we observed a tendency to increase the deposition of collagen I and decrease collagen III in the animals that received treatment, although these differences were not significant.

The imbalance in MMP-9 activity leads to an increase in the deposition of extracellular matrix proteins, including collagen, resulting in fibrosis (135). Junger et al. (93) showed that late treatment with hypertonic, as well as activating neutrophils, increased the release of elastases, leading to increased tissue damage. Thus, our findings show that the increase in MMP-9 expression in the tissue may be triggering tissue damage and, consequently, changes in collagen deposition.

As we saw in the results of the early hypertonic treatment, collagen deposition is related to the increase in FAK expression in response, possibly, to the increase in neutrophils and nitric oxide synthesis. We therefore quantified this protein and the agents involved in its activation pathway in order to confirm the action of the hypertonic solution.

We observed that late treatment with volume replacement increased nitric oxide synthesis and, consequently, FAK activation in lung tissue, which could be related to increased collagen deposition in the tissue. These results are in line with our findings of an increase in the deposition of type I collagen, showing that treatment with hypertonic would prevent the replacement of the more elastic collagen III by collagen I, which would be responsible for the decrease in lung function.

As expected, the respiratory mechanics parameters followed the results of collagen deposition in the tissue. Although we observed a tendency for the resistance and elastance of the tissue to increase, the results were not significantly different. The region of the lung parenchyma is where the greatest deposition of collagen is observed and this deposition is an event described as directly related to the loss of lung function (127, 136).

Thus, these results emphasize the current line of conduct in intensive care of treatment as early as possible, suggesting that late treatment could increase the need for mechanical ventilation in patients with ARDS as a result of sepsis, leading to a worsening prognosis for these patients (34, 137).

CONCLUSIONS

6. Conclusions

• Early treatment with hypertonic solution prevented mortality in endotoxemic rats, reducing tissue damage and collagen deposition in the lung tissue of endotoxemic animals 24 hours after treatment, inhibiting the FAK pathway possibly due to a decrease in nitric oxide production.

• The pulmonary mechanics of the animals induced to endotoxemia and/or treated 15 minutes after induction of the disease showed a decrease in resistance and elastance in the lung tissue when compared to the animals treated with hypertonic solution.

• Late treatment, carried out 1.5 hours after induction of the disease, proved to be harmful, as it did not prevent mortality and led to lung tissue damage, through an increase in the expression and activity of MMP-9 and an imbalance in the deposition of type I and type III collagens.

• When administered late, the hypertonic solution failed to favorably modulate the FAK pathway induced by nitric oxide, increasing pulmonary fibrosis and, consequently, worsening lung mechanics parameters.

• Our results show two fundamental aspects of hypertonic solution: the pathway of action of early treatment with hypertonic solution on lung remodeling through FAK inhibition and the therapeutic window of hypertonic solution. This last aspect may explain the difficulty found in reproducing the beneficial effects of treatment with hypertonic solution in patients, showing that the time of administration of hypertonic solution is crucial for its therapeutic action.

REFERENCES

7. References

1. Silva E, Pedro Mde A, Sogayar AC, Mohovic T, Silva CL, Janiszewski M, et al. Brazilian Sepsis Epidemiological Study (BASES study). Crit Care. 2004 Aug;8(4):R251-60.

2. Abraham E, Matthay MA, Dinarello CA, Vincent JL, Cohen J, Opal SM, et al. Consensus conference definitions for sepsis, septic shock, acute lung injury, and acute respiratory distress syndrome: time for a reevaluation. Crit Care Med. 2000 Jan;28(1):232-5.

3. Angus DC, Linde-Zwirble WT, Lidicker J, Clermont G, Carcillo J, Pinsky MR. Epidemiology of severe sepsis in the United States: analysis of incidence, outcome, and associated costs of care. Crit Care Med. 2001 Jul;29(7):1303-10.

4. Dellinger RP, Levy MM, Rhodes A, Annane D, Gerlach H, Opal SM, et al. Surviving Sepsis Campaign: international guidelines for management of severe sepsis and septic shock, 2012. Intensive Care Med. 2012 Feb;39(2):165-228.

5. Cipolle MD, Pasquale MD, Cerra FB. Secondary organ dysfunction. From clinical perspectives to molecular mediators. Crit Care Clin. 1993 Apr;9(2):261-98.

6. Parker MM, Shelhamer JH, Bacharach SL, Green MV, Natanson C, Frederick TM, et al. Profound but reversible myocardial depression in patients with septic shock. Ann Intern Med. 1984 Apr;100(4):483-90.

7. Parker MM, Ognibene FP, Parrillo JE. Peak systolic pressure/end-systolic volume ratio, a load-independent measure of ventricular function, is reversibly decreased in human septic shock. Crit Care Med. 1994 Dec;22(12):1955-9.

8. Bohuslav J, Kravchenko VV, Parry GC, Erlich JH, Gerondakis S, Mackman N, et al. Regulation of an essential innate immune response by the p50 subunit of NF-kappaB. J Clin Invest. 1998 Nov 1;102(9):1645-52.

9. Moore FA, Moore EE, Read RA. Postinjury multiple organ failure: role of extrathoracic injury and sepsis in adult respiratory distress syndrome. New Horiz. 1993 Nov;1(4):538-49.

10. Bone RC. Sepsis, the sepsis syndrome, multi-organ failure: a plea for comparable definitions. Ann Intern Med. 1991 Feb 15;114(4):332-3.

11. Christians ES, Yan LJ, Benjamin IJ. Heat shock factor 1 and heat shock proteins:

Critical partners in protection against acute cell injury. Crit Care Med. 2002 Jan;30(1 Supp):S43-S50.

12. Salvo I, de Cian W, Musicco M, Langer M, Piadena R, Wolfler A, et al. The Italian SEPSIS study: preliminary results on the incidence and evolution of SIRS, sepsis, severe sepsis and septic shock. Intensive Care Med. 1995 Nov;21 Suppl 2:S244-9.

13. Vincent JL. Update on sepsis: pathophysiology and treatment. Acta Clin Belg. 2000 Mar-Apr;55(2):79-87.

14. Pollack M, Ohl CA. Endotoxin-based molecular strategies for the prevention and treatment of gram-negative sepsis and septic shock. Curr Top Microbiol Immunol. 1996;216:275-97.

15. Grinnell BW, Joyce D. Recombinant human activated protein C: a system modulator of vascular function for treatment of severe sepsis. Crit Care Med. 2001 Jul;29(7 Suppl):S53-60; discussion S-1.

16. João Andrade L. Sales Júnior CMD, Rodrigo Hatum, Paulo César S. P. Souza, André Japiassù,, Cleovaldo T. S. Pinheiro GF, Odin Barbosa da Silva, Mariza D'Agostino Dias, Edwin Koterba,, Fernando Suparregui Dias CP. Sepsis Brazil: Epidemiological Study of Sepsis in Brazilian Intensive Care Units. Revista Brasileira Terapia Intensiva. 2006;18:9-17.

17. van den Berghe G, Wouters P, Weekers F, Verwaest C, Bruyninckx F, Schetz M, et al. Intensive insulin therapy in the critically ill patient. N Engl J Med. 2001 Nov 8;345(19):1359-67.

18. Rivers E, Nguyen B, Havstad S, Ressler J, Muzzin A, Knoblich B, et al. Early goal-directed therapy in the treatment of severe sepsis and septic shock. N Engl J Med. 2001 Nov 8;345(19):1368-77.

19. Annane D. Glucocorticoids in the treatment of severe sepsis and septic shock. Curr Opin Crit Care. 2005 Oct;11(5):449-53.

20. Cao C, Matsumura K, Yamagata K, Watanabe Y. Involvement of cyclooxygenase-2 in LPS-induced fever and regulation of its mRNA by LPS in the rat brain. Am J Physiol. 1997 Jun;272(6 Pt 2):R1712-25.

21. Medzhitov R, Janeway C, Jr. Innate immunity. N Engl J Med. 2000 Aug 3;343(5):338-44.

22. Medzhitov R, Janeway CA, Jr. An ancient system of host defense. Curr Opin Immunol. 1998 Feb;10(1):12-5.

23. Skidmore BJ, Chiller JM, Morrison DC, Weigle WO. Immunologic properties of bacterial lipopolysaccharide (LPS): correlation between the mitogenic, adjuvant, and immunogenic activities. J Immunol. 1975 Feb;114(2 pt 2):770-5.

24. Strieter RM, Kunkel SL, Bone RC. Role of tumor necrosis factor-alpha in disease states and inflammation. Crit Care Med. 1993 Oct;21(10 Suppl):S447- 63.

25. Medzhitov R, Janeway C, Jr. Innate immune recognition: mechanisms and pathways. Immunol Rev. 2000 Feb;173:89-97.

26. Kaisho T, Akira S. Dendritic-cell function in Toll-like receptor- and MyD88-knockout mice. Trends Immunol. 2001 Feb;22(2):78-83.

27. Marshall R, Bellingan G, Laurent G. The acute respiratory distress syndrome: fibrosis in the fast lane. Thorax. 1998 Oct;53(10):815-7.

28. Cinel I, Dellinger RP. Advances in pathogenesis and management of sepsis. Curr Opin Infect Dis. 2007 Aug;20(4):345-52.

29. Soriano FG, Nogueira AC, Caldini EG, Lins MH, Teixeira AC, Cappi SB, et al. Potential role of poly(adenosine 5'-diphosphate-ribose) polymerase activation in the pathogenesis of myocardial contractile dysfunction associated with human septic shock. Crit Care Med. 2006 Apr;34(4):1073-9.

30. Vincent JL, Sun Q, Dubois MJ. Clinical trials of immunomodulatory therapies in severe sepsis and septic shock. Clin Infect Dis. 2002 Apr 15;34(8):1084-93.

31. Rietschel ET, Brade H, Holst O, Brade L, Muller-Loennies S, Mamat U, et al. Bacterial endotoxin: Chemical constitution, biological recognition, host response, and immunological detoxification. Curr Top Microbiol Immunol. 1996;216:39-81.

32. Wheeler AP, Bernard GR. Treating patients with severe sepsis. N Engl J Med. 1999 Jan 21;340(3):207-14.

33. Matsuda N, Hattori Y. Systemic inflammatory response syndrome (SIRS): molecular pathophysiology and gene therapy. J Pharmacol Sci. 2006 Jul;101(3):189-98.

34. Christensen VB, Nielsen JS, Tonnesen EK. [Sepsis in the critically-ill patient]. Ugeskr Laeger. 2007 Feb 19;169(8):703-5.

35. Chung TP, Laramie JM, Province M, Cobb JP. Functional genomics of critical illness and injury. Crit Care Med. 2002 Jan;30(1 Suppl):S51-7.

36. Delves PJ, Roitt IM. The immune system. Second of two parts. N Engl J Med. 2000

Jul 13;343(2):108-17.

37. Philippart F, Cavaillon JM. Sepsis mediators. Curr Infect Dis Rep. 2007 Sep;9(5):358-65.

38. Jean-Baptiste E. Cellular mechanisms in sepsis. J Intensive Care Med. 2007 Mar-Apr;22(2):63-72.

39. Balibrea JL, Arias-Diaz J. Acute respiratory distress syndrome in the septic surgical patient. World J Surg. 2003 Dec;27(12):1275-84.

40. Rojas M, Woods CR, Mora AL, Xu J, Brigham KL. Endotoxin-induced lung injury in mice: structural, functional, and biochemical responses. Am J Physiol Lung Cell Mol Physiol. 2005 Feb;288(2):L333-41.

41. Martin GS, Eaton S, Mealer M, Moss M. Extravascular lung water in patients with severe sepsis: a prospective cohort study. Crit Care. 2005 Apr;9(2):R74-82.

42. Guo RF, Ward PA. Role of oxidants in lung injury during sepsis. Antioxid Redox Signal. 2007 Nov;9(11):1991-2002.

43. Murao Y, Loomis W, Wolf P, Hoyt DB, Junger WG. Effect of dose of hypertonic saline on its potential to prevent lung tissue damage in a mouse model of hemorrhagic shock. Shock. 2003 Jul;20(1):29-34.

44. Uhlig S, Brasch F, Wollin L, Fehrenbach H, Richter J, Wendel A. Functional and fine structural changes in isolated rat lungs challenged with endotoxin ex vivo and in vitro. Am J Pathol. 1995 May;146(5):1235-47.

45. Czermak BJ, Breckwoldt M, Ravage ZB, Huber-Lang M, Schmal H, Bless NM, et al. Mechanisms of enhanced lung injury during sepsis. Am J Pathol. 1999 Apr;154(4):1057-65.

46. Barbarin V, Nihoul A, Misson P, Arras M, Delos M, Leclercq I, et al. The role of pro- and anti-inflammatory responses in silica-induced lung fibrosis. Respir Res. 2005;6:112.

47. Torry DJ, Richards CD, Podor TJ, Gauldie J. Anchorage-independent colony growth of pulmonary fibroblasts derived from fibrotic human lung tissue. J Clin Invest. 1994 Apr;93(4):1525-32.

48. Suki B, Ito S, Stamenovic D, Lutchen KR, Ingenito EP. Biomechanics of the lung parenchyma: critical roles of collagen and mechanical forces. J Appl Physiol. 2005 May;98(5):1892-9.

49. Buttenschoen K, Kornmann M, Berger D, Leder G, Beger HG, Vasilescu C.

Endotoxemia and endotoxin tolerance in patients with ARDS. Langenbecks Arch Surg. 2008 Jul;393(4):473-8.

50. Santos FB, Nagato LK, Boechem NM, Negri EM, Guimaraes A, Capelozzi VL, et al. Time course of lung parenchyma remodeling in pulmonary and extrapulmonary acute lung injury. J Appl Physiol. 2006 Jan;100(1):98-106.

51. Wei W, Ma B, Li HY, Jia Y, Lv K, Wang G, et al. Biphasic effects of selective inhibition of transforming growth factor beta1 activin receptor-like kinase on LPS-induced lung injury. Shock. Feb;33(2):218-24.

52. Vittal R, Horowitz JC, Moore BB, Zhang H, Martinez FJ, Toews GB, et al. Modulation of prosurvival signaling in fibroblasts by a protein kinase inhibitor protects against fibrotic tissue injury. Am J Pathol. 2005 Feb;166(2):367-75.

53. Cox BD, Natarajan M, Stettner MR, Gladson CL. New concepts regarding focal adhesion kinase promotion of cell migration and proliferation. J Cell Biochem. 2006 Sep 1;99(1):35-52.

54. Mian MF, Kang C, Lee S, Choi JH, Bae SS, Kim SH, et al. Cleavage of focal adhesion kinase is an early marker and modulator of oxidative stress- induced apoptosis. Chem Biol Interact. 2008 Jan 10;171(1):57-66.

55. Lagares D, Busnadiego O, Garcia-Fernandez RA, Kapoor M, Liu S, Carter DE, et al. Inhibition of focal adhesion kinase prevents experimental lung fibrosis and myofibroblast formation. Arthritis Rheum. 2012 May;64(5):1653-64.

56. Petroni RC, Teodoro WR, Guido MC, Barbeiro HV, Abatepaulo F, Theobaldo MC, et al. Role of focal adhesion kinase in lung remodeling of endotoxemic rats. Shock. 2012 May;37(5):524-30.

57. Pelosi P, Rocco PR, Negrini D, Passi A. The extracellular matrix of the lung and its role in edema formation. An Acad Bras Cienc. 2007 Jun;79(2):285- 97.

58. Vanlaere I, Libert C. Matrix metalloproteinases as drug targets in infections caused by gram-negative bacteria and in septic shock. Clin Microbiol Rev. 2009 Apr;22(2):224-39, Table of Contents.

59. Kahari VM, Saarialho-Kere U. Matrix metalloproteinases and their inhibitors in tumor growth and invasion. Ann Med. 1999 Feb;31(1):34-45.

60. Tandon A, Sinha S. Structural insights into the binding of MMP9 inhibitors. Bioinformation.5(8):310-4.

61. Davey A, McAuley DF, O'Kane CM. Matrix metalloproteinases in acute lung injury: mediators of injury and drivers of repair. Eur Respir J. Oct;38(4):959-70.

62. Parks WC, Wilson CL, Lopez-Boado YS. Matrix metalloproteinases as modulators of inflammation and innate immunity. Nat Rev Immunol. 2004 Aug;4(8):617-29.

63. Corbel M, Boichot E, Lagente V. Role of gelatinases MMP-2 and MMP-9 in tissue remodeling following acute lung injury. Braz J Med Biol Res. 2000 Jul;33(7):749-54.

64. Muhs BE, Patel S, Yee H, Marcus S, Shamamian P. Increased matrix metalloproteinase expression and activation following experimental acute pancreatitis. J Surg Res. 2001 Nov;101(1):21-8.

65. Arkovitz MS, Wispe JR, Garcia VF, Szabo C. Selective inhibition of the inducible isoform of nitric oxide synthase prevents pulmonary transvascular flux during acute endotoxemia. J Pediatr Surg. 1996 Aug;31(8):1009-15.

66. Nathan C. Nitric oxide as a secretory product of mammalian cells. FASEB J. 1992 Sep;6(12):3051-64.

67. Parratt JR. Nitric oxide in sepsis and endotoxaemia. J Antimicrob Chemother. 1998 Jan;41 Suppl A:31-9.

68. Titheradge MA. Nitric oxide in septic shock. Biochim Biophys Acta. 1999 May 5;1411(2-3):437-55.

69. Numata M, Suzuki S, Miyazawa N, Miyashita A, Nagashima Y, Inoue S, et al. Inhibition of inducible nitric oxide synthase prevents LPS-induced acute lung injury in dogs. J Immunol. 1998 Mar 15;160(6):3031-7.

70. Rice TW, Bernard GR. Therapeutic intervention and targets for sepsis. Annu Rev Med. 2005;56:225-48.

71. Riedemann NC, Guo RF, Ward PA. Novel strategies for the treatment of sepsis. Nat Med. 2003 May;9(5):517-24.

72. Shih CC, Chen SJ, Chen A, Wu JY, Liaw WJ, Wu CC. Therapeutic effects of hypertonic saline on peritonitis-induced septic shock with multiple organ dysfunction syndrome in rats. Crit Care Med. 2008 Jun;36(6):1864-72.

73. Staudenmayer KL, Maier RV, Jelacic S, Bulger EM. Hypertonic saline modulates innate immunity in a model of systemic inflammation. Shock. 2005 May;23(5):459-63.

74. Roch A, Guervilly C, Papazian L. Fluid management in acute lung injury and ards. Ann

Intensive Care. 2011;1(1):16.

75. Wiedemann HP, Wheeler AP, Bernard GR, Thompson BT, Hayden D, deBoisblanc B, et al. Comparison of two fluid-management strategies in acute lung injury. N Engl J Med. 2006 Jun 15;354(24):2564-75.

76. Hagiwara S, Iwasaka H, Hidaka S, Hishiyama S, Noguchi T. Danaparoid sodium inhibits systemic inflammation and prevents endotoxin-induced acute lung injury in rats. Crit Care. 2008;12(2):R43.

77. Velasco IT, Pontieri V, Rocha e Silva M, Jr, Lopes OU. Hyperosmotic NaCl and severe hemorrhagic shock. Am J Physiol. 1980 Nov;239(5):H664-73.

78. Junger WG, Coimbra R, Liu FC, Herdon-Remelius C, Junger W, Junger H, et al. Hypertonic saline resuscitation: a tool to modulate immune function in trauma patients? Shock. 1997 Oct;8(4):235-41.

79. Oliveira RP, Velasco I, Soriano F, Friedman G. Clinical review: Hypertonic saline resuscitation in sepsis. Crit Care. 2002 Oct;6(5):418-23.

80. Oliveira RP, Velasco I, Soriano FG, Friedman G. Clinical review: Hypertonic saline resuscitation in sepsis. Crit Care. 2002 Oct;6(5):418-23.

81. Wade C, Grady J, Kramer G. Efficacy of hypertonic saline dextran (HSD) in patients with traumatic hypotension: meta-analysis of individual patient data. Acta Anaesthesiol Scand Suppl. 1997;110:77-9.

82. Wade CE, Grady JJ, Kramer GC. Efficacy of hypertonic saline dextran fluid resuscitation for patients with hypotension from penetrating trauma. J Trauma. 2003 May;54(5 Suppl):S144-8.

83. Wade CE, Grady JJ, Kramer GC, Younes RN, Gehlsen K, Holcroft JW. Individual patient cohort analysis of the efficacy of hypertonic saline/dextran in patients with traumatic brain injury and hypotension. J Trauma. 1997 May;42(5 Suppl):S61-5.

84. Wade CE, Kramer GC, Grady JJ, Fabian TC, Younes RN. Efficacy of hypertonic 7.5% saline and 6% dextran-70 in treating trauma: a meta-analysis of controlled clinical studies. Surgery. 1997 Sep;122(3):609-16.

85. Mattox KL, Maningas PA, Moore EE, Mateer JR, Marx JA, Aprahamian C, et al. Prehospital hypertonic saline/dextran infusion for post-traumatic hypotension. The U.S.A. Multicenter Trial. Ann Surg. 1991 May;213(5):482-91.

86. Ciesla DJ, Moore EE, Biffl WL, Gonzalez RJ, Silliman CC. Hypertonic saline

attenuation of neutrophil cytotoxic response is reversed hypertonic challenge. Surgery. 2001;129:567-75.

87. Orlic T, Loomis WH, Shreve A, Namiki S, Junger WG. Hypertonicity increases cAMP in PMN and blocks oxidative burst by PKA-dependent and - independent mechanisms. Am J Physiol Cell Physiol. 2002 Jun;282(6):C1261- 9.

88. Kramer G, Elgjo G, Poli de Figueiredo LF, Wade C. HYPEROSMOTIC-HYPERONCOTIC SOLUTIONS. Clinical Anesthesiology. 1997;11:147-60.

89. Rizoli SB, Kapus A, Fan J, Li YH, Marshall JC, Rotstein OD. Immunomodulatory effects of hypertonic resuscitation on the development of lung inflammation following hemorrhagic shock. J Immunol. 1998 Dec 1;161(11):6288-96.

90. Powers KA, Woo J, Khadaroo RG, Papia G, Kapus A, Rotstein OD. Hypertonic resuscitation of hemorrhagic shock upregulates the antiinflammatory response by alveolar macrophages. Surgery. 2003 Aug;134(2):312-8.

91. Papia G, Burrows LL, Sinnadurai S, Marshall JC, Tawadros PS, Kapus A, et al. Hypertonic saline resuscitation from hemorrhagic shock does not impair the neutrophil response to intraabdominal infection. Surgery. 2008 Nov;144(5):814-21.

92. Rizoli SB, Kapus A, Parodo J, Rotstein OD. Hypertonicity prevents lipopolysaccharide-stimulated CD11b/CD18 expression in human neutrophils in vitro: role for p38 inhibition. J Trauma. 1999 May;46(5):794-8; discussion 8-9.

93. Junger WG, Hoyt DB, Davis RE, Herdon-Remelius C, Namiki S, Junger H, et al. Hypertonicity regulates the function of human neutrophils by modulating chemoattractant receptor signaling and activating mitogen-activated protein kinase p38. J Clin Invest. 1998 Jun 15;101(12):2768-79.

94. Yu G, Chi X, Hei Z, Shen N, Chen J, Zhang W, et al. Small volume resuscitation with 7.5% hypertonic saline, hydroxyethyl starch 130/0.4 solution and hypertonic sodium chloride hydroxyethyl starch 40 injection reduced lung injury in endotoxin shock rats: comparison with saline. Pulm Pharmacol Ther. 2012 Feb;25(1):27-32.

95. Kim HW, Breiding P, Greenburg AG. Enhanced modulation of hypotension in endotoxemia by concomitant nitric oxide synthesis inhibition and nitric oxide scavenging. Artif Cells Blood Substit Immobil Biotechnol. 1997 Jan- Mar;25(1-2):153-62.

96. Pfaffl MW. A new mathematical model for relative quantification in realtime RT-PCR. Nucleic Acids Res. 2001 May 1;29(9):e45.

97. Livak KJ, Schmittgen TD. Analysis of relative gene expression data using real-time quantitative PCR and the 2(-Delta Delta C(T)) Method. Methods. 2001 Dec;25(4):402-8.

98. Shi DW, Zhang J, Jiang HN, Tong CY, Gu GR, Ji Y, et al. LPS pretreatment ameliorates multiple organ injuries and improves survival in a murine model of polymicrobial sepsis. Inflamm Res. Sep;60(9):841-9.

99. Chapman HA. Disorders of lung matrix remodeling. J Clin Invest. 2004 Jan;113(2):148-57.

100. Liu W, Shan LP, Dong XS, Liu XW, Ma T, Liu Z. Effect of early fluid resuscitation on the lung in a rat model of lipopolysaccharide-induced septic shock. Eur Rev Med Pharmacol Sci. 2013 Jan;17(2):161-9.

101. Thiel M, Buessecker F, Eberhardt K, Chouker A, Setzer F, Kreimeier U, et al. Effects of hypertonic saline on expression of human polymorphonuclear leukocyte adhesion molecules. J Leukoc Biol. 2001 Aug;70(2):261-73.

102. Powers KA, Zurawska J, Szaszi K, Khadaroo RG, Kapus A, Rotstein OD. Hypertonic resuscitation of hemorrhagic shock prevents alveolar macrophage activation by preventing systemic oxidative stress due to gut ischemia/reperfusion. Surgery. 2005 Jan;137(1):66-74.

103. Gurfinkel V, Poggetti RS, Fontes B, da Costa Ferreira Novo F, Birolini D. Hypertonic saline improves tissue oxygenation and reduces systemic and pulmonary inflammatory response caused by hemorrhagic shock. J Trauma. 2003 Jun;54(6):1137-45.

104. Zhu GC, Quan ZY, Shao YS, Zhao JG, Zhang YT. [The study of hypertonic saline and hydroxyethyl starch treating severe sepsis]. Zhongguo Wei Zhong Bing Ji Jiu Yi Xue. Mar;23(3):150-3.

105. Chopra A, Kumar V, Dutta A. Hypertonic versus normal saline as initial fluid bolus in pediatric septic shock. Indian J Pediatr. Jul;78(7):833-7.

106. Imm A, Carlson RW. Fluid resuscitation in circulatory shock. Crit Care Clin. 1993 Apr;9(2):313-33.

107. Villa P, Sartor G, Angelini M, Sironi M, Conni M, Gnocchi P, et al. Pattern of cytokines and pharmacomodulation in sepsis induced by cecal ligation and puncture compared with that induced by endotoxin. Clin Diagn Lab Immunol. 1995 Sep;2(5):549-53.

108. Keck T, Balcom JHt, Fernandez-del Castillo C, Antoniu BA, Warshaw AL. Matrix metalloproteinase-9 promotes neutrophil migration and alveolar capillary leakage in pancreatitis-associated lung injury in the rat. Gastroenterology. 2002 Jan;122(1):188-201.

109. Davey A, McAuley DF, O'Kane CM. Matrix metalloproteinases in acute lung injury: mediators of injury and drivers of repair. Eur Respir J. 2011 Oct;38(4):959-70.

110. Dooley JL, Abdel-Latif D, St Laurent CD, Puttagunta L, Befus D, Lacy P. Regulation of inflammation by Rac2 in immune complex-mediated acute lung injury. Am J Physiol Lung Cell Mol Physiol. 2009 Dec;297(6):L1091-102.

111. Dos Santos CC. Advances in mechanisms of repair and remodelling in acute lung injury. Intensive Care Med. 2008 Apr;34(4):619-30.

112. Rocco PR, Negri EM, Kurtz PM, Vasconcellos FP, Silva GH, Capelozzi VL, et al. Lung tissue mechanics and extracellular matrix remodeling in acute lung injury. Am J Respir Crit Care Med. 2001 Sep 15;164(6):1067-71.

113. Faffe DS, Seidl VR, Chagas PS, Goncalves de Moraes VL, Capelozzi VL, Rocco PR, et al. Respiratory effects of lipopolysaccharide-induced inflammatory lung injury in mice. Eur Respir J. 2000 Jan;15(1):85-91.

114. Clemente CF, Tornatore TF, Theizen TH, Deckmann AC, Pereira TC, Lopes-Cendes I, et al. Targeting focal adhesion kinase with small interfering RNA prevents and reverses load-induced cardiac hypertrophy in mice. Circ Res. 2007 Dec 7;101(12):1339-48.

115. Cai GQ, Zheng A, Tang Q, White ES, Chou CF, Gladson CL, et al. Downregulation of FAK-related non-kinase mediates the migratory phenotype of human fibrotic lung fibroblasts. Exp Cell Res. May 15;316(9):1600-9.

116. Guido MC CC, Moretti AI, Barbeiro HV, Debbas V, Caldini EG, Franchini KG, Soriano FG. Small Interfering RNA target focal adhesion kinase prevents cardiac dysfunction in endotoxemia. shock. 2011:Epub ahead of print.

117. Siesser PM, Hanks SK. The signaling and biological implications of FAK overexpression in cancer. Clin Cancer Res. 2006 Jun 1;12(11 Pt 1):3233-7.

118. Hsia DA, Mitra SK, Hauck CR, Streblow DN, Nelson JA, Ilic D, et al. Differential regulation of cell motility and invasion by FAK. J Cell Biol. 2003 Mar 3;160(5):753-67.

119. Hsu YC, Wang LF, Chien YW. Nitric oxide in the pathogenesis of diffuse pulmonary fibrosis. Free Radic Biol Med. 2007 Mar 1;42(5):599-607.

120. Maa MC, Chang MY, Li J, Li YY, Hsieh MY, Yang CJ, et al. The iNOS/Src/FAK axis is critical in Toll-like receptor-mediated cell motility in macrophages. Biochim Biophys Acta. 2010 Jan;1813(1):136-47.

121. Yuan SY, Shen Q, Rigor RR, Wu MH. Neutrophil transmigration, focal adhesion kinase

and endothelial barrier function. Microvasc Res. 2012 Jan;83(1):82-8.

122. Vo PA, Lad B, Tomlinson JA, Francis S, Ahluwalia A. Autoregulatory role of endothelium-derived nitric oxide (NO) on Lipopolysaccharide-induced vascular inducible NO synthase expression and function. J Biol Chem. 2005 Feb 25;280(8):7236-43.

123. Poli-de-Figueiredo LF, Cruz RJ, Jr., Sannomiya P, Rocha ESM. Mechanisms of action of hypertonic saline resuscitation in severe sepsis and septic shock. Endocr Metab Immune Disord Drug Targets. 2006 Jun;6(2):201-6.

124. Tsushima K, King LS, Aggarwal NR, De Gorordo A, D'Alessio FR, Kubo K. Acute lung injury review. Intern Med. 2009;48(9):621-30.

125. Faffe DS, Zin WA. Lung parenchymal mechanics in health and disease. Physiol Rev. 2009 Jul;89(3):759-75.

126. Costa EL, Schettino IA, Schettino GP. The lung in sepsis: guilty or innocent? Endocr Metab Immune Disord Drug Targets. 2006 Jun;6(2):213-6.

127. Leite-Junior JH, Garcia CS, Souza-Fernandes AB, Silva PL, Ornellas DS, Larangeira AP, et al. Methylprednisolone improves lung mechanics and reduces the inflammatory response in pulmonary but not in extrapulmonary mild acute lung injury in mice. Crit Care Med. 2008 Sep;36(9):2621-8.

128. Vincent JL, Gottin L. Type of fluid in severe sepsis and septic shock. Minerva Anestesiol. 2011 Dec;77(12):1190-6.

129. Shih CC, Tsai MF, Chen SJ, Tsao CM, Ka SM, Huang HC, et al. Effects of small-volume hypertonic saline on acid-base and electrolytes balance in rats with peritonitis-induced sepsis. Shock. 2012 Dec;38(6):649-55.

130. Gao J, Zhao WX, Xue FS, Zhou LJ, Yu YH, Zhou HB. Effects of different resuscitation fluids on acute lung injury in a rat model of uncontrolled hemorrhagic shock and infection. J Trauma. 2009 Dec;67(6):1213-9.

131. van Haren FM, Sleigh J, Boerma EC, La Pine M, Bahr M, Pickkers P, et al. Hypertonic fluid administration in patients with septic shock: a prospective randomized controlled pilot study. Shock. 2011 Mar;37(3):268-75.

132. Inoue Y, Chen Y, Pauzenberger R, Hirsh MI, Junger WG. Hypertonic saline up-regulates A3 adenosine receptor expression of activated neutrophils and increases acute lung injury after sepsis. Crit Care Med. 2008 Sep;36(9):2569-75.

133. Murao Y, Hoyt DB, Loomis W, Namiki S, Patel N, Wolf P, et al. Does the timing of

hypertonic saline resuscitation affect its potential to prevent lung damage? Shock. 2000 Jul;14(1):18-23.

134. Hashiguchi N, Lum L, Romeril E, Chen Y, Yip L, Hoyt DB, et al. Hypertonic saline resuscitation: efficacy may require early treatment in severely injured patients. J Trauma. 2007 Feb;62(2):299-306.

135. Gueders MM, Foidart JM, Noel A, Cataldo DD. Matrix metalloproteinases (MMPs) and tissue inhibitors of MMPs in the respiratory tract: potential implications in asthma and other lung diseases. Eur J Pharmacol. 2006 Mar 8;533(1-3):133-44.

136. Davidson KG, Bersten AD, Barr HA, Dowling KD, Nicholas TE, Doyle IR. Endotoxin induces respiratory failure and increases surfactant turnover and respiration independent of alveolocapillary injury in rats. Am J Respir Crit Care Med. 2002 Jun 1;165(11):1516-25.

137. Wiersinga WJ, van der Poll T. [Sepsis: new insights into its pathogenesis and treatment]. Ned Tijdschr Geneeskd.154:A1130.

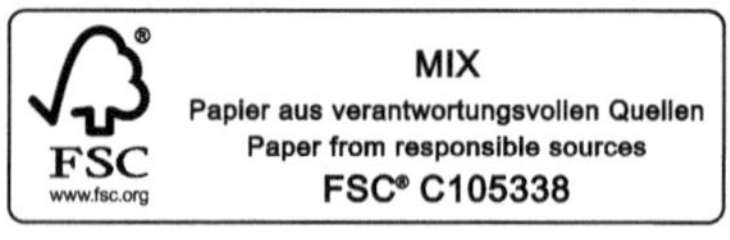

Printed by Books on Demand GmbH, Norderstedt / Germany